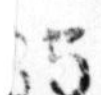

Natural Fertility Awareness

Natural Fertility Awareness

A Practical Guide to the Natural Achievement or Avoidance of Conception

by John & Farida Davidson

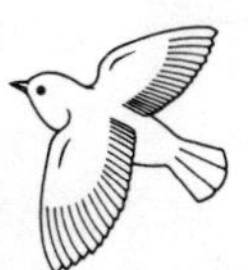

SAFFRON WALDEN
THE C. W. DANIEL COMPANY LIMITED

First published in Great Britain in 1986
by The C. W. Daniel Company Limited
1 Church Path, Saffron Walden,
Essex, CB10 1JP, England

ISBN 0 85207 175 2

Designed by Tina Dutton
Production in association with
Book Production Consultants, Cambridge
Typeset by Cambridge Photosetting Services in Bembo
Printed and bound by Billings, Worcester

Contents

Acknowledgements

We would like to thank all who have contributed to our knowledge of these subjects, in particular Dr. Anna Flynn and her colleagues from the Birmingham Maternity Hospital, the Alive Polarity Fellowship in the U.S.A., where Farida first studied these methods, and all those who are researching, teaching and writing about their discoveries and experiences. We are just one more link in this expanding chain.

The drawings are by Alan Bailey of Cambridge.

Foreword

by

Dr Anna Flynn F.R.C.O.G.

Dr. Anna Flynn, an obstetrician and gynaecologist with a natural bent of mind, is one of the world's foremost researchers into the natural indicators of fertility, having also conducted research on this subject for the World Health Organization. She is one of the founder members of Britain's National Association of Natural Family Planning Teachers.

Nature, which is said never to forgive, is finally demanding retribution for the physical abuses inflicted on mankind by mankind over the recent past decades, through the use of artificial methods of contraception. This fact is driving our sophisticated western societies to seek a more natural system of birth control without increased health risks. The rapid scientific developments, however, that are leading many people to flee the tyrany of disharmonious technology, have also brought to mankind a more profound understanding of fertility with beneficial repercussions on natural ways of controlling it. As a consequence, the last decade has witnessed the publication of more books about Natural Family Planning and Fertility Awareness than the preceding fifty years. This book is a further valuable contribution to that bibliography.

In more ways than one John and Farida Davidson are 'Naturals', so it is not surprising that they should write a book about Natural Fertility Awareness. In common with some previous publications, this book contains a description of the basic physiological facts required to enable couples to assess their fertility in a natural way. However, it also offers some additional information.

Since John was, until recently, a Cambridge University computer professional, it also seems 'natural' that he should enlist the aid of the computer to help couples wishing to use Natural Birth Control. The innovatory character of the book lies in its introduction of the small computer-based instrument (*Ovia*) which enables couples to objectivise and automatically assess their fertile and infertile phases. Many couples born into and brought up in our modern age will feel more secure at having a cross-check (as it were) to tell them when sexual intercourse may result in a pregnancy and this is just what *Ovia* does. Since no harmful drugs or devices have to be introduced into the body, the method is still quite natural.

I believe that this book will appeal to and help all those who seek to understand natural bodily rhythms and I can thoroughly recommend it.

Dr. Anna M. Flynn F.R.C.O.G.
Birmingham Maternity Hospital
October 1985

General Introduction

Reading through the history of man's understanding of the fertile times in a woman's reproductive cycle, one is immediately struck by two factors. Firstly, that it is essentially a man's understanding: all doctors who have made their mark on this history have, until recent, more enlightened times, been men. Secondly, that mostly they got it completely wrong!

In order to understand a thing, we bring into play our intellect, our intuition and most importantly, our experience. A man is forever debarred from experiencing what it is to have a woman's body. Only in the most close empathetic of relationships with his wife or long-term partner, can a man begin to understand the subtleties of how a woman feels about her body. It will always be outside his experience (and vice versa): only a woman can really know what makes a woman tick! So it is not surprising that the most infertile times of a cycle have, historically, been variously ascribed to every part of the cycle, not infrequently including what we now know to be those most fertile times.

Similarly, it is only in recent times that women have started writing in women's terms about feminine emotions and psychology. The old style of women's liberation often meant the masculinization of the women in order that they might make their way in a working world dominated by men. More modern approaches realize the beauty, strength and necessity of the feminine principle in nature, with women and men working together as equal partners, each with their own role to play in the economy of the cosmos.

In some ancient cultures, more in tune with the natural rhythms of nature, fertility awareness and understanding appears to have been practised, based not so much on our 20th century analytical knowledge, but on a more feminine, intuitive understanding and in harmony with the cycles of heaven and earth. The over-analytical, scientific approach, while clearly having its advantages, tears apart the delicate fabric of intuitive understanding, and our ability to live out of synchronization with nature puts us at a distance from a simple and natural way of being.

We cannot, of course, turn back the clock, neither would we want to. What is needed, however, is to establish the principle of harmony between our technology and ourselves. If man is to survive into the twenty-first century, he has to re-arrange and re-assess his technology. Technology and science should work for us, for the general benefit of the human race. Selfish aspects must be identified and harmonized. We must endeavour to be far-sighted and caring in regard to our planet and its peoples.

This is not, of course, a book on environmental care and keeping a pleasant planet, but the aspect that concerns us here is that of an expanding world population and how to keep it in check, without recourse to drugs, the Pill, devices or surgery all with negative aspects psychologically, emotionally or physically.

Modern research, largely by women doctors, into the scientific, hormone controlling sequence of a woman's cycle has given us some invaluable indicators as to the changing patterns of fertility and infertility within that cycle, that are totally in harmony with nature and which encourage the inner growth and flow of energy so necessary for the inner development of a whole and complete human being.

We believe that this wonderful knowledge will bring much relief to millions of women in the world, struggling with pills, devices in their wombs, sterilization, sperm-killing foams, time release capsules implanted in their skins and the Lord only knows what else! It is the aim of this book to lay out this information clearly for all to understand, regardless of their level of education or ability to grasp scientific detail. We hope that it will help men and women move with more natural ease into the 21st century.

John Davidson M.A. Cantab
Cambridge, 1985

Introduction – Woman to Woman

It is very hard to find your way as a woman in these modern times. There are so many influences and pressures. We are not a part of a culture which shows us the way with myth, metaphor, tradition and ritual. We do not have any rites of initiation which pass on the wisdom of our mothers and our mothers' mothers.

Each woman must find her own path, and either live as a reflection of the expectation of others, or develop her interior, intuitive wisdom and instinct which will guide her to know what is right. That is perhaps the most difficult thing to do, and yet recovering that inborn feminine nature will prove a centre of strength in a confusing and changing world.

We cannot rely on external sources of information, no matter how authoratative they are, to guide us as to what is right. That has been proven again and again with the side-effects of drugs such as thalidomide, the Pill and other synthesized medicine. We pay the price. Our only means of protection is to tune into our inner knowing. Our body will then tell us what is right.

In my natural medicine practice of over twelve years, I have taken thousands of case histories and counselled so many women patients. The same message is made clear again and again: the path to a healthy female body lies in understanding your own strengths and weaknesses (we use Iridology as a tool to give us an insight into the workings of all the parts of the body and its systems and how they interrelate). It is necessary to keep the body clean and clear by activating all the eliminative channels (the bowels, lymph, kidneys, lungs and skin), to eat a nutritious diet containing a high proportion of fruits, vegetables, grains, nuts and seeds, to have a stable emotional life and wise moderate living habits. While it is true that life creates stress and unexpected events and our archetypal patterns lead us into destinies and reactions which create health problems, it is the work of maturity to learn to ride the waves of life so that our bodies serve us well.

The signs of illness are there far in advance for a woman to recognize if she chooses. However, many woman shrug these aside due to the pressures of family and work responsibilities, and in ignorance and fear. These signs, once set in motion, increase until a chronic disease pattern emerges. It then requires major efforts to undo the complex of mind/emotion/body which forms the knot of the disease. For the women who accept surgery, most bring a tale of woe that they have never felt the same since. While surgery does become a life preserving necessity if the situation is allowed to build into a threatening state, *the approach to women's medicine should be that of prevention and preservation*. We must learn how to keep our bodies well.

Much of what threatens women is centred around the reproductive system. Methods of contraception, birth practices and radical surgery are great stress areas for women. We have become dependent on a technology which we fear, resist and do not understand. How can we find the way out, the way back to wisdom and understanding? How can we make our bodies our own again?

The first step is to feel, to listen, to pay attention. When you notice any changes note them down. Observe yourself. Look for changes in bowels and urine, lines on the face, pains, tiredness. The moment a change comes, sit down, centre on that and seek understanding.

Deal with things immediately, when they occur. If you do not they will grow into major imbalances which will take much time, attention and professional help to undo.

Seek support groups. Find women of like mind and meet regularly. Read books together and talk about them. Invite speakers to your group. Attend lectures and weekend seminars. Try various disciplines in alternative medicine until you have a network of communication through which you can seek help, support and assistance when any imbalance has become so strong that you cannot change it on your own.

Know that your life is a progression. Even if you have not had older women of wisdom to teach and guide you, you can learn by experience and when your children are grown, you can serve as a guiding light for other women, teaching them what you have learned and helping them on their way. Your mature years will have a purpose and vision to which you can look forward.

The communication network is expanding every year. We are creating a new reality. If you read the history of medicine in such fine books as *Green Pharmacy* by Barbara Griggs, you will see that the term, "the weaker sex" came because of hundreds of years of mercurial and arsenic medication for every common female complaint, as well as purging and copious bleeding. Eventually, many women became near-invalids and certainly needed the sheltered life which was their social role at that time. Now we are finding our way back to our strength. We have the right to healthy and fulfilled lives and we need to unite and share our knowledge, so that we can create the future together.

Natural Fertility Awareness is one of the great methods by which we can gain our conscious freedom from harmful, dubious and damaging products which not only harm our bodies but create problems for future generations. Loving cooperation between men and women, giving full respect to the female body in its sacred aspect as the womb of creation, provides the ambience for a loving relationship free of fear, resentment and domination/submission games. Together the partners participate in harmonious unity, using all the body's signs, working with nature's cycles and honouring the sacred aspects of both the masculine and feminine principles.

Whether your purpose is to achieve or avoid conception, conscious participation in Natural Fertility Awareness will lift your sexuality out of ignorance and confusion into intelligent and sensitive harmony with nature. All of your life, you will receive benefit and the world of your body, and the world you live in will reflect this harmony and intelligence.

Natural Fertility Awareness provides the opportunity for a merging of the instinctive, intuitive wisdom of nature and woman with the logical, scientific order of mind and the masculine principle. While we are all made of both masculine and feminine, containing both within us, this acceptance and harmonious interchange of these energies centred in the sexual and procreative areas will contribute respect and appreciation during loving communion. As partners you will share a close attunement to each other's needs.

It gives me great happiness to participate in this project and see it launched in the world at this time. I offer my gratitude and admiration for all my husband has done towards this great service to women and mankind. This union of body wisdom and intelligent logic has created a new methodology for the 21st century, the best of a harmony between science and nature.

Farida Davidson
Cambridge, 1985

CHAPTER I

The Fertility Cycle

The essential, natural purpose behind the fertility cycle is the preparation of the womb or uterus to receive a fertilized ovum and for pregnancy and childbirth to ensue. If conception does not take place, then the preparation of the tissues is reversed (menstruation) and a new cycle of preparation begins. So that all events take place in their correct order, the body has a remarkable series of chemical triggers, known as hormones. It is these hormones which govern the state and condition of the various organs and body tissues involved in the reproductive process. The contraceptive hormone pill, for example, works by interfering with this cycle, maintaining these reproductive organs and tissues in a condition in which pregnancy cannot occur.

The cycle is continuous, but for the purposes of explanation, it may be considered as consisting of four phases:

→ Menstruation → Pre-Ovulation → Ovulation → Post-Ovulation ↩

Some authorities describe the cycle as consisting of three phases relating to the relative fertility of that part of the cycle. Thus we have:

→ Pre-Ovulatory Infertile Phase → Pre-Ovulatory Fertile Phase → Post-ovulatory Infertile Phase ↩

In this later description, ovulation occurs during the fertile phase, with menstruation being included in the pre-ovulatory phase.

Bear in mind that:

1. Ovulation can only happen once during a cycle, approximately two weeks before the following period. The hormonal sequence and development of the follicle or envelope in which the ovum is produced does not permit otherwise. Fraternal twins may occur if a second ovulation takes place, but this can only be within twenty-four hours of the first ovulation. Identical twins are caused by a division of the fertilized ovum, before implantation in the uterine wall.
2. The lifetime of an ovum is normally six to twelve hours, with an outside limit of twenty four hours.
3. The lifetime of sperm can be a maximum of five days, depending upon conditions within the vagina and cervix, and the seminal fluid itself.

It is thus very clear that pregnancy can only occur within five or six days during a cycle, allowing for the joint lifetimes of both sperm and ovum.

Therefore, the whole art of fertility awareness is deciding, before it happens, when ovulation is going to take place.

CHAPTER 2

The Controlling Hormone Sequence

It is not at all essential that you understand or remember the hormonal controlling sequence of the fertility cycle in order to practise *Natural Fertility Awareness* methods. However, if you can take the time to understand the basic principles, you will find that the fertility cycle and its indicators make a more complete picture. Nor is it necessary to be able to recall all the details of the reproductive organs and their physiology, yet if you understand them, even just a little, you may find that the relevant facts fall into place more readily.

Having said which, if you decide to skip this short chapter, the gaps in your knowledge will not prevent you from understanding and practising the contents of the remainder of the book. It is just that we feel it ought to be here for those who want to know about it. And we have ourselves found this knowledge very helpful.

The Reproductive System

Firstly we need to look at the women's reproductive system, (see figures 1, 2 and 3), the drawings being simplified to show only those organs which relate directly to the reproductive system.

There are two further organs that need to be considered, these are the endocrine (hormone secreting) glands situated in the brain: the *pituitary* and the *hypothalamus*. The pituitary is a master controller endocrine gland that plays a major part in the overall organization and control of the total hormonal or endocrine system. The hypothalamus is the environment and stress monitor and communicates such factors to the pituitary gland through its biochemical, hormone triggers.

Relating our description of their functions to the

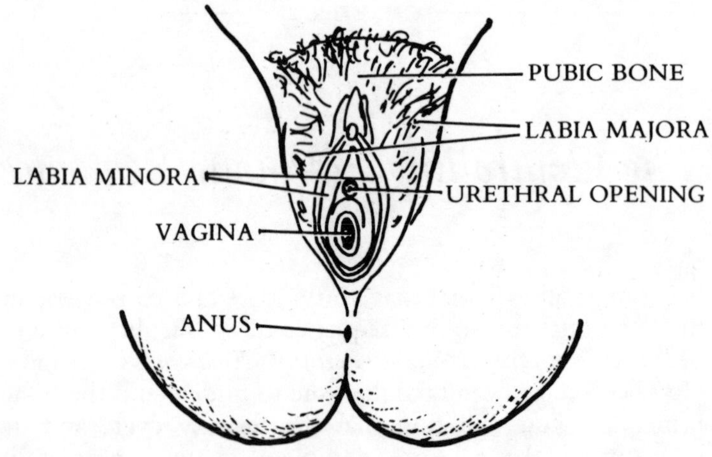

Figure 1 – The Womans External Sexual Organs

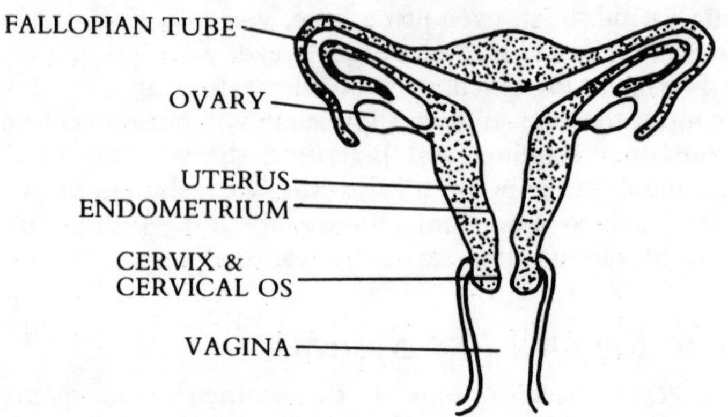

Figure 2 – The Womans Reproductive Anatomy (frontal cross-section)

hormone sequence, the story goes like this; starting immediately *after* menstruation has finished:

1. Firstly, the pituitary secretes *Follicle Stimulating Hormone* (FSH), which acts on the *ovaries* to stimulate a small number of the ovarian *follicles* to produce the hormone *oestrogen*. The follicles are the protective envelopes within the ovary which actually produce one *ovum* each, the ovum being the female egg.

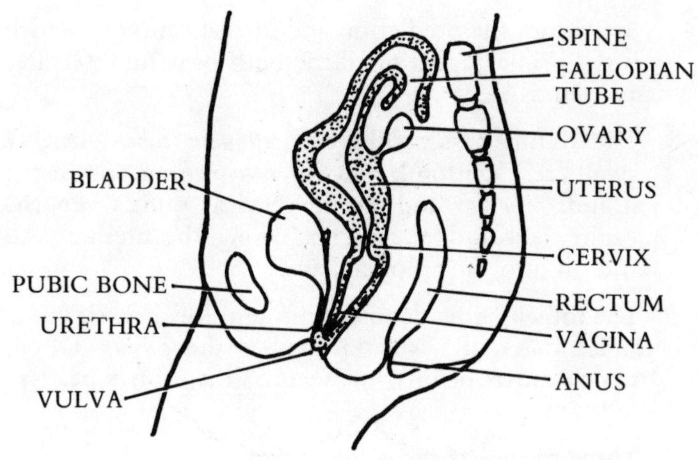

Figure 3 – The Womans Reproductive Anatomy (side view)

2. Of these follicles, only one or occasionally two, will develop to maturity in each cycle. As the follicles develop, so the oestrogen level builds-up, and is secreted by the follicle itself. Four of the effects of *oestrogen* are:
   (a) The pituitary FSH production is inhibited, thus suppressing the maturation of other follicles.
   (b) The *uterine* wall, the *endometrium,* starts to thicken in preparation for receiving a fertilized ovum. The *uterus* or *womb* is where the unborn child develops during pregnancy.
   (c) The *cervical glands* are stimulated to produce *mucus* that is nourishing and friendly towards *sperm,* while the cervical aperture, the *os,* opens to permit the passage of the mucus downwards and the sperm upwards.
   (d) The uterine supporting muscles contract, raising the position of the *cervix* within the *vagina.*
3. The oestrogen level continues to build up until it reaches a point where the pituitary gland is stimulated to produce a surge of *Luteinizing Hormone* (LH), lasting for only a few days.
4. Within four to sixty-four hours LH stimulates the follicle, to open up and release the ovum. This is

ovulation, the prediction and identification of which is the primary goal of all methods of natural fertility awareness.

5. The ovum passes into the *fallopian tube* where it awaits fertilization by sperm, swimming within the strands of wet and fertile cervical mucus, up the vagina, through the cervix, along the uterine wall and on into the fallopian tube.

6. The follicle, now devoid of its egg, forms itself into a small mass of tissue known as the *corpus luteum,* which now begins to secrete the hormone *progesterone.*

7. Three of the effects of *progesterone* are:
   (a) The pituitary is inhibited from producing further LH or FSH. *No further ovulation can thus take place during this cycle.*
   (b) The cervical os closes and/or is plugged by thick mucus which is both hostile to sperm and prevents its passage. At the same time, the uterine supporting muscles relax and the cervix falls lower into the vagina.
   (c) There is a small rise in the basal body temperature, the temperature of the undisturbed body at rest.

8. The ovum now passes down the fallopian tube and if fertilized, it implants itself into the thick and nourishing uterine wall where it begins to develop. Progesterone continues to be produced during the early stages of pregnancy, but is later replaced by other pregnancy hormones.

9. If fertilization does not take place, then the corpus luteum begins to degenerate and, with the falling level of progesterone, the uterine wall breaks down and is shed, at *menstruation.*

10. At the same time, the drop in progesterone concentration allows the pituitary to once more begin production of FSH; the temperature then falls, and the cycle starts all over again.

Other Effects of Female Hormones

There is a close connection between the emotional and mental life and the levels of oestrogen and progesterone in a woman and similarly with the corresponding male hormone, testosterone, in a man.

These hormones are also responsible for the maintenance of the secondary sexual characteristics – breast tissue, body hair, psychological aspects and so on. But the internal biochemical interactions linked to the hormonal sequence are far from being fully understood. We discuss this in relation to the Pill in a later chapter, but suffice it to say here that we are not at all convinced that interfering with some of the key biochemical triggers in our bodies is of long-term benefit to us, although the short-term, self-interested gain is very clear.

And we are not alone in this thinking. There are at present getting on for 200,000 women practising natural methods of birth control in the United Kingdom. This means nearly half a million people, including their partners, or more than one in fifty of the adult population of child-bearing age. The publication of three or four books on the subject within the last two years, by British publishers alone, bears witness to the growing interest. *Natural Fertility Awareness* is really worth investigating.

Hormone	Source	Main effects
FSH	Pituitary	• Stimulates ovarian oestrogen production
Oestrogen	Ovarian follicles Corpus luteum	• High levels inhibit pituitary FSH secretion • Endometrium thickens • Cervix ripens, opens and rises • Cervix produces fertile mucus • Secondary sexual characteristics maintained
LH	Pituitary	• LH surge stimulated by high oestrogen levels • Stimulates ovulation within normally 12 hours, outside limit is 64 hours • Promotes formation of corpus luteum
Progesterone	Corpus luteum	• Causes a rise in BBT • Inhibits pituitary FSH release • Endometrium softens • Cervix closes and lowers • Infertile mucus produced

Figure 4 – The Hormonal Sequence and Interactions

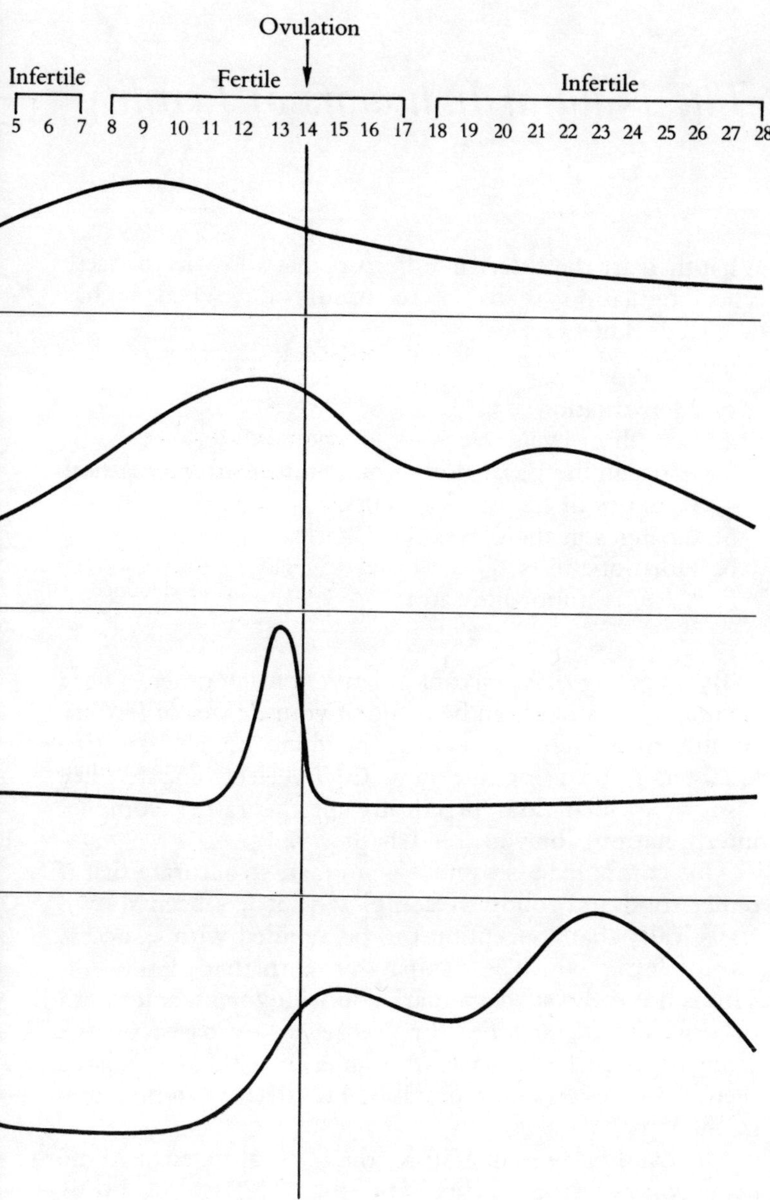
Ovulation
Infertile
Fertile
Infertile
5 6 7 8 9 10 11 12 13 14 15 16 17 18 19 20 21 22 23 24 25 26 27 28

CHAPTER 3

The Natural Indicators of Fertility

What then are the external indicators that allow us to assess when ovulation is likely to occur and when it has occurred? They are:

1. Menstruation
2. Length of cycle
3. A rise in the Basal Body Temperature after ovulation
4. Changes in the cervical mucus
5. Changes in the cervix itself
6. Hormone tests
7. Various minor indicators

By assessing these factors, relative to each other, a very accurate assessment can be made of your degree of fertility or infertility. This can either be done on a chart (see Chapter 7) or using the new *OVIA* electronic fertility assessor, which does practically all the rather complex interpretations for you (see Chapter 8).

This combined assessment is, in fact, so accurate that if understood and followed completely, it has been shown statistically that conception can be avoided with a success rate of 99%, which is comparable with that of the Pill. This is not really such a remarkable achievment, since both the Pill and *Natural Fertility Awareness* are based on the same hormonal sequence. A sequence that, as we have seen is both exact and repeatable. Full details can be found in chapter 9.

The basal body temperature, the cervical mucus and the condition of the cervix are the THREE MAJOR INDICATORS described more fully in Chapters 4, 5, and 6

1. *Menstruation*

In the early part of the cycle, the uterine wall or *endometrium* thickens and is generally prepared for a possible pregnancy. Like a good gardener lovingly preparing the soil for his plants or seeds, nature prepares the womb for a possible fertilized ovum. If fertilization does not take place, this endometrium softens, finally breaking down and being shed at the time of menstruation. Thus, unless a woman has a history of short cycles, during menstruation and in the few days afterwards, conception is highly unlikely to occur. The first day of the period is generally taken as day one of the cycle, because it is so clearly defined and noticeable.

Reports of pregnancy due to making love during a period are normally tracable to mid-term bleeding or spotting lasting usually for only a day or so and by no means as heavy as a period. This mid-term bleeding is due to changes in the hormone levels and can occur at the peak of the fertile time, just as ovulation is about to take place. It does not occur with all women, but you do need to be aware of it. The basic rule is always: *if in doubt – don't!* We discuss this bleeding in greater depth at the end of this chapter.

2. *The Length of the Cycle and The Rhythm Method*

The length of the cycle has historically been used, with notably disastrous results, as a means of attempting to calculate when ovulation will take place. Generally speaking, the length of time between ovulation and the commencement of a period, will be between 12 to 16 days. However, the length of the pre-ovulatory phase can and does vary. With a cycle length of the average twenty eight days, the pre-ovulatory phase, including your period, will also be around 12 to 16 days. Nevertheless, with a very short cycle of 21 days, ovulation will occur around days 5 to 9, while with an extra long cycle of 40 days, ovulation will have occured between days 24 and 28.

With sperm capable of living up to five days it is clear that pregnancy is possible even when making love during your period. Since it is not apparent in advance when ovulation is likely to occur, relying on the rhythm method alone means it is easy to get caught out by an early ovulation and thus become pregnant.

Some people feel, although there is no evidence yet identified, that ovulation can perhaps be triggered by making love. This would seem to be unlikely, since the ovum must mature and conditions in the vagina, cervix and uterus must also be ready to receive the fertilized egg. However, if making love when ovulation is imminent anyway, could bring ovulation forward, then again the rhythm method would fail, while the other indicators would have given a clear picture of your state of fertility.

The only way in which the rhythm method can be used with any degree of success is to know the shortest of your last six to twelve cycles, then use the following calculation:

Shortest cycle minus 21 equals the last safe, infertile day

So if you have had a shortest cycle of 21, then there are no safe days!.

Similarly, if you assume that ovulation must be over because of the length of time since your last period, you can again run into trouble. Ovulation can be delayed by stress, travelling, emotional upsets and shocks, etc., and may not have occurred even when you think that your period is due any day.

It is easy to see, therefore, how the unpredictability of ovulation based on calendar calculations, combined with the difficulty of long periods of enforced abstinence, can lead to pregnancy, when using this method alone.

What is needed are day by day indicators that are reflective of the current state of the reproductive system and are sensitive to changes such as stress, travelling and so on.

3. *The Basal Body Temperature*

Now we come to the first of the three major indices of fertility. The Basal Body Temperature or BBT is the temperature of the body at rest, unaffected by activity, food or drink. In practice, this means your temperature on waking in the morning, before you get out of bed.

Without becoming too technical, the hormone progesterone, produced after ovulation increases the BBT by about 0.2°C or 0.4°F. This rise is sudden and normally quite easily identifiable, giving one an accurate indication that ovulation has taken place. This indicates the post-ovulatory infertile phase where the chances of becoming pregnant have been shown to be less than 1 in a 100.

Full details of how to be sure that you have correctly identified this shift are given in the next chapter.

4. *Cervical Mucus*

As the ovum is nearing ripeness and the uterine lining is prepared for conception, so too does the cervix make preparation for fertilization to take place. The cervix, you will recall from the previous chapter, is the part at the base of the uterus that projects downwards into the vagina. In essence, the mucus produced by the cervix becomes moist and then wet and can normally be detected at the opening of the vagina.

5. *The Condition of the Cervix*

Just as the cervical mucus changes as ovulation approaches, so too does the condition of the cervix. It becomes soft, like a ripening fruit and moves higher up into abdomen. At the same time, the cervical opening into the vagina enlarges, permitting the flow of wet, lubricative and fertile mucus, within which the spermatazoa can swim up to meet with and fertilize the ovum.

6. *Hormone Tests*

All the external indicators are linked to the levels of the reproductive hormones, in particular oestrogen, progesterone and the Luteinizing Hormone (LH). These hormones are found in the blood stream and their metabolites or breakdown-compounds are also to be found in the urine. A number of pharmaceutical companies are endeavouring to produce simple, domestic, urine dipstick tests to identify the infertile phases of a cycle and while their research on these tests is meeting with some success, their introduction as a generally available and well-tested product is probably some years away. The difficulty is that they attempt to measure the relative levels of oestrogen and progesterone in the urine, levels which vary from person to person and from cycle to cycle.

However, there is a domestic urine test for the Luteinizing Hormone, the hormone that triggers ovulation. This is a tremendous help to those with infertility problems. One of the causes of infertility is cycles in which there is no ovulation – *anovulatory* cycles. This means that if, for example, only one cycle in six produced an ovum, then there would only be about five or six days, probably less, in six months, when conception could occur. The temperature indicators will tell you if ovulation has occurred in a cycle, but by that time, it is too late. The mucus and cervical conditions can help too, but the LH test will give a highly accurate indicator of imminent ovulation. So then is the time to try for pregnancy!

7. *Minor Indicators*

In addition to the more obvious indicators of where in her cycle a woman may be, there are a number of less obvious signs which once understood can be taken as valuable secondary confirmation. These are, however, not experienced by every woman.

Ovulation Pain. Towards the middle of the cycle, almost certainly connected with the events immediately surrounding ovulation itself, some women feel a sharp pain lasting for a few hours or a dull, more diffuse ache lasting for longer, up to a day or two. There are a number of theories regarding its origin. However, since it occurs low down in the abdomen, in the vicinity of the left or right ovary, it is assumed to be a result either of the slight rupturing of the ovary as the egg is released or to changes in the fallopian tube.

Mid-Cycle Bleeding, also called Breakthrough Bleeding or Spotting. A blood-tinged vaginal discharge can occur mid-cycle originating from the top layers of the endometrium, due to changes in the hormone levels. This is of infrequent occurrence, but it is important to be aware of it since it can occur around the time of greatest fertility. The rule is that if no temperature shift has been recorded then any bleeding should be considered as mid-cycle until it is certain that it is a period. You should also consider any such bleeding as suspect if the mucus and/or cervical signs are simultaneously indicating that you are fertile.

Breast Feelings. Both oestrogen and progesterone quite commonly produce symptoms of soreness, tenderness or heaviness in the breasts. The soreness is generally associated with high levels of oestrogen and therefore with fertility, while heaviness is associated with progesterone and hence with the post-ovulatory infertile phase.

Emotional Changes. Depression, a lack of, or an increase in energy, tiredness, irritability, waxing and waning of sexual desire and many other shades of mood are quite regularly experienced rhythmically, keeping pace with the changing cycle. These vary from person to person and one can simply note one's own variations on the theme. It is all a part of being a woman and a knowledge that these moods have a physiological aspect can help both women and their partners come to terms with their ups and downs.

Dr. Anna Flynn, from Birmingham Maternity Hospital, one of the world's leading researchers in Natural Family Planning, once commented on the number of women in their mid-twenties that she sees, coming off the Pill for the first time since puberty. In effect, this means that they have never experienced one of the main aspects of being a woman. The results are understandably traumatic. Interfering with nature will always produce side-effects of one kind or another. It is a part of the intrinsic law of cause and effect that governs all interplay amongst the energy patterns of the physical universe.

Human Aspects

You might think, if you have never tried it, that taking your temperature and observing mucus signs every day could become a chore and make the whole thing bigger then you want it to be. In fact, the reverse is found to be true. It is no more a chore than brushing your hair or noting the weather conditions when deciding which clothes to wear. Moreover, the knowledge it gives of body cycles and the increased sharing, co-operation and intimacy it can bring between partners is of inestimable, value.

The quality of life is not measured by having a quick and easy, but superficial, manner of disposing of its problems, but by those indefinable qualities that go towards the making of mature and wholesome humanity. Being in harmony with yourself, with nature and with your partner, not putting unwholesome substances into one's body, taking clear-headed (well – reasonably clear!) responsibility for the quality of one's life – all these contribute, along with many other factors, towards one's growth as a human being.

The use of natural fertility awareness will only be considered by those seeking a higher manner of expression as a human being. Others will be happy with a symptomatic and superficial approach to both birth control, and being alive generally.

CHAPTER 4

The Three Major Indicators – Basal Body Temperature

When To Take It?

The Basal Body Temperature is the body temperature at rest, unaffected by activity, food or drink. In practise, this means your temperature at the same waking time each day before getting out of bed. Some authorities suggest that it is all right to put the thermometer in your mouth and then proceed to get up and move about for the necessary five minutes to register your temperature. This is probably fine but you would need to check it works for you. You should do this by taking your temperature before getting up and noting the reading, then having shaken the thermometer down slip it back into your mouth while you start dressing or whatever. Check it again after five minutes to see if there is any differences from the first reading. Do this on several mornings and if there is no difference, then this method is all right for you. The main thing is to be consistent about the time, to within half an hour or less.

If you have had a disturbed night, perhaps the children have kept you up, then it is essential that you have been asleep for at least an hour before waking at your regular time, to take your temperature; and that you have had at least three hours sleep.

Advantages and Disadvantages

Taking your temperature each morning and recording it, is something that anyone can start with right away. It is the easiest to learn of the three main fertility indicators. The temperature shift when it comes, is quite apparent and it means that you can immediately make use of the post-ovulatory infertile phase for making unprotected love, with a contraceptive certainty of about 99%. It immediately puts you into contact with your natural rhythm and cycle. It is also quite exciting to see the theory coming to life in your own practice.

If you can encourage your partner to become involved as a part of his shared responsibility then that is an excellent idea. Some husbands even take their wife's temperature themselves and keep the record for her, making their own assessment from the chart or handling the input to the *OVIA* fertility assessor.

The disadvantages of using the temperature shift *on its own* is that ovulation is detected retrospectively and it is hence of little use in achieving pregnancy in couples with infertility difficulties. Some doctors advise their patients with infertility problems to look for a temperature shift as an indication of ovulation, without pointing out that by that time, it is most probably already too late for conception within that cycle.

A friend of ours who had been trying for many years to become pregnant was told to take her temperature and look for the shift, but since no detailed instructions were given on what to do or what to look for, she soon lost heart. She had no idea of the right way of doing it or what she was really looking for or that even if detected, the temperature shift would not help her much. Fortunately, the story has a happy ending, because they now have a large and bouncy, one year old and hope that another will follow in the not too distant future. But the first one took them ten years.

The other disadvantage of using the temperature indicator alone is that it cannot indicate the infertile days in the early part of the cycle and therefore requires longer periods of abstinence than when using the combined methods. This required abstinence may, in itself, be too much for some couples, resulting in unplanned pregnancies. If adhered to, however, the method on its own is highly reliable, normally rated at 99%.

The Temperature Shift

The hormone progesterone – produced by the *corpus luteum*, the structure formed out of the ovarian follicle after the release of the ovum – induces a rise in the basal body temperature of about 0.2°C or 0.4°F. This shift is quite marked and readily detected even amongst normal small variations in the body temperature. To be completely sure that you have detected the post-ovulatory progesterone-induced shift, a simple rule of thumb has been worked out, which is as follows:

The post-ovulatory infertile phase begins on the third morning of a sustained temperature shift, all three of which are greater than any of the temperatures recorded on the previous six days.

The rise will usually be at least 0.2°C or 0.4°F between the highest of the low six and the lowest of the next three. *(See chart 2).*

The only exception to the rule is that any obvious 'spike' in the low six temperatures can be ignored *(see chart 3).* Furthermore, the first four temperatures of a cycle should be ignored since the temperature may still be coming down from the previous cycle, *(see chart 2).*

If you are plotting your temperature on a chart, you should be able to draw a *cover line* above the six lower temperatures and below the three higher ones, *(see chart 2).*

A very few women have a consistent temperature shift of only 0.3°F/0.15°C, but the pattern should be readily observable. Only work to this kind of shift when you have seen it consistently over two or three cycles.

It is also fairly common to see a small drop of about 0.05°C/0.1°F immediately before the temperature rise, often coinciding with *Peak Mucus* (see chapter 5).

How to Take Your Temperature

Firstly, you need a thermometer with an expanded scale over the lower range of body temperatures (35°–39°C/96°–100°F instead of 35°–42°C/94°–108°F). This means either a glass and mercury fertility thermometer or an electronic digital thermometer. There is a new one, recently introduced, which has an accuracy to two decimal places of degrees Celsius (Centigrade) and to one decimal place in degrees Fahrenheit.

Be sure that any fertility thermometer you purchase has easily readable divisions to at least 0.05°C/0.1°F.

It is a good idea to have two thermometers in case you break or lose one of them. However, since thermometers can vary by as much as 0.1°C/0.2°F, you should calibrate your spare against your normal thermometer. Then, should you need to change thermometers mid-cycle, you must adjust each temperature according to any difference, before recording it.

The procedure is as follows:

1. Shake down your thermometer the evening before or after your last recording, so as to be ready for the morning. Leave it somewhere handy, at your bedside. You should shake it with a quick flick of the wrist, rather like cracking a whip, preferably over something soft like your bed, in case you drop it or hit something! Digital thermometers, of course, don't need shaking down.

2. Upon waking, and at the time decided, take your temperature. You can take your temperature either orally, rectally or vaginally. Having decided which place to use you should stick to it for a complete cycle, because the rectal and vaginal temperatures are higher than the mouth. If you use your mouth, then the glass tube containing the mercury goes *underneath your tongue* for at least five minutes to allow your mouth to reach body temperature as well as the thermometer. If you are using a digital thermometer, then you need to keep your mouth shut for at least three to five minutes before inserting the thermometer, the reading normally being complete within a minute. if using the vaginal or rectal routes, then do be careful not to put it in too far and don't break it! And don't fall asleep again with the thermometer in place! About three minutes will be a long enough time, except for the digital thermometer which takes a minute. The digital thermometer is rather neat, in that the digits continue to flash until it has reached its stable temperature.

3. You now need to record your temperature either on a chart or using *OVIA* (see chapters 7 & 8), but unless you are using the digital thermometer which turns itself off after a few minutes, you can leave the thermometer at your bedside until you are ready to

read it. As long as you don't put it in a warm spot – a radiator or a sunny window-sill, for example – a glass and mercury thermometer will retain its exact temperature until you shake it down again. The digital thermometer has an automatic switch off after a few minutes, so you need to keep a pen and pad or your chart handy.

4. Wash the thermometer in cold water only.

Finally, a few do's and don'ts. Don't drink anything just prior to taking your temperature orally. If your oral temperatures are irregular, then try taking it one of the other ways. If there is any doubt about the reading, round it down rather than up. If the thermometer gets chilled at night in a cold bedroom, warm it up against your cheek first – if you put it straight into its place, it could cool the place down and give you an incorrect reading. And if you suspect that you have an increased temperature due to illness, don't use a fertility thermometer or it may go off the scale and you could break it.

Disturbances to Your Temperature

There are a number of factors which may cause disturbances to the basal body temperature, (*see charts 4 and 5*). Normally, these are readily identifiable and as long as you record the probability of a disturbance and there are not too many of them, they cause no problems in interpretation. They will normally appear as an obvious spike on a chart and can simply be ignored. The following factors are known to cause temperature fluctuations:

Early or Late Rising
Illness
Emotional Upset, Shock, Stress, Over-excitement
Travel, especially across time zones
Changing Hours of Shift Work
Disturbed nights
Alcohol and drugs.

Early or Late Rising. Your BBT rises by between 0.05°C/ 0.1°F and 0.15°C/0.3°F for each hour later that you take your waking temperature, between 5 a.m. and 11 a.m.

Having fixed your own standard time for temperature taking, if you deviate from this, you will need to make an adjustment. The lowest rise is normally about 0.05°C/0.1°F and if you have not checked your own pattern, then use this adjustment as the safest option if ever you rise more than half an hour earlier or later than usual. However, it is really best to find a chance to lie in one morning, taking your temperature at intervals of half an hour, to see how much it changes. If the change is of the order of 0.02°C/0.05°F per hour, then you can ignore it anyway, unless you are several hours away from your usual time.

The spring and autumn daylight saving change of timing will, for a short while, have the same effect as sleeping in or getting up early. It takes about two or three days to adjust to the new rhythm.

Illness. Naturally, if you have a cold, 'flu or something worse, then your temperature pattern will show an increase. However, it is always readily distinguishable from the small sustained rise after ovulation, (*see chart 4*).

Emotional Upset, Shock, Stress, Over-excitement. Two factors are at work here. Firstly, upsets and shock may cause a brief rise in your BBT which you should record along with your temperature. Secondly, periods of stress may be reflected in delayed ovulation and subsequent long cycles. This is nature's way of planning pregnancies for times when you can cope with it. These times without menstruation may even span over a number of years as evidenced by the now well-known cases of women in concentration camps; with a return to regular cycles after the stress has passed. The danger as regards temperature recording to discover the post-ovulatory infertile phase is, that one might be tempted to think that the fertile phase has passed, simply because of the length of time elapsed since your last period. So the rule of three temperatures higher than the previous six temperatures, together with the 0.2°C/0.4°F shift, *must* be adhered to. It is here, also, that cross-checking with the cervical mucus and cervix indicators can be of great help, (*see chart 4*).

Travel and Shift Work, Late Nights. Any upset to your normal 24 hour, circadian rhythm will disturb your temperature to a greater or lesser extent. After an air-flight across time-zones, it may take a week to settle down and if it happens at a critical point in your cycle, obscuring any potential temperature shift, you may need to wait until your next period until you are sure again where you are. Alternatively, the travel may delay ovulation, so don't take chances in a cycle which may turn out to be longer than usual.

Similarly with shift work, when you change shifts, there is likely to be an upset if it disturbs your sleeping hours. So don't assume that you have had a temperature shift if the information could have been caused by other factors. Remember that the post-ovulatory temperature rise is *sustained*, so even if there is a disturbance during the shift, the three over six rule will still apply if you ignore the suspect readings in your addition, i.e. you may need to take four days instead of three if one of them is disturbed, (*see chart 4*).

Alcohol and Drugs. Finally, even a glass or two of alcohol the night before, can induce a small temperature rise and you should record the temperature as potentially disturbed, especially if a rise is noticed. Most medicinal drugs do not influence your BBT, but there are so many available that you should be aware of this possibility and check it for yourself. Aspirin and some other pain-killers may cause a drop in temperature. Medicines containing reproductive hormones will definitely influence the cycle and most probably the temperature, so that none of the natural fertility indicators can be relied upon.

Ovulation and the Temperature Shift

Researchers into the exact timing of ovulation in relation to the temperature rise have used both hormone tests and ultrasound techniques to identify a ruptured ovarian follicle developing into the corpus luteum. It seems that ovulation can occur up to five days before and two days after the shift, giving a potential fertility span of about thirteen days – five days for long-life sperm, seven days during which ovulation can occur plus one day for the life of the ovum, if it occurs two days after the shift.

Anovulatory cycles are quite distinctive, (*see chart 9*). The temperature rambles on and on, often over a long cycle of 30 to 40 or more days, never indicating any temperature shift.

Pregnancy and the Temperature Shift

As the level of the hormone progesterone begins to drop immediately prior to menstruation, so too does your BBT, the fall perhaps taking a further four days after menstruation has begun to reach the lower pre-ovulatory level. If your temperature stays high for twenty days or longer, you may well be pregnant, (*see chart 10*). This is the earliest indicator of pregnancy other than your own intuition. If you have been keeping a record, then you will be able to know almost exactly when conception occurred. The formula to calculate the date of probable birth is:

Date of temperature shift minus 7 plus 9 calendar months.

And may we wish you a happy and fulfilled nine months! This can be a time of great emotional happiness and joy.

CHAPTER 5

The Three Major Indicators – Cervical Mucus

Of the three main fertility indicators, the cervical mucus and cervix signs provide the information for fertility assessment in the early part of the cycle, while the temperature shift gives us an exact indication of the beginning of the post-ovulatory infertile phase. So taking an extremely safe calendar calculation to assess the start of the pre-ovulatory infertile phase, double or triple checked against the mucus and cervix indicators, we end up with a method of birth control which surveys prove to be better than 99% safe.

The cervical mucus, backed up by cervix observations and the LH urine test, if there are infertility problems, is the most effective indicator to predicting ovulation and the easiest method to learn. It has none of the disadvantages associated with laboratory tests, and you can see it day-by-day in your own home, or wherever you happen to be.

The cervical mucus indicators, first pioneered by Drs John and Evelyn Billings, must, however, be well-learnt and if you have any doubts about your observations you should consult a Natural Family Planning teacher or a friend who knows the methods thoroughly and is not too shy to tell you exactly what to look for. Since so much is at stake, it is really worthwhile spending the necessary time becoming fully aquainted with all the ins and outs of a knowledge which will last you a lifetime and is something you can teach to others as well as to your children.

The Role of Cervical Mucus in the Fertility Cycle

Under the control, once again, of the hormone sequence, this time mostly oestrogen, the cervical mucus has an important role to play in the fertility cycle, while at the same time providing us with the second of the Three Major Natural Indicators of Fertility.

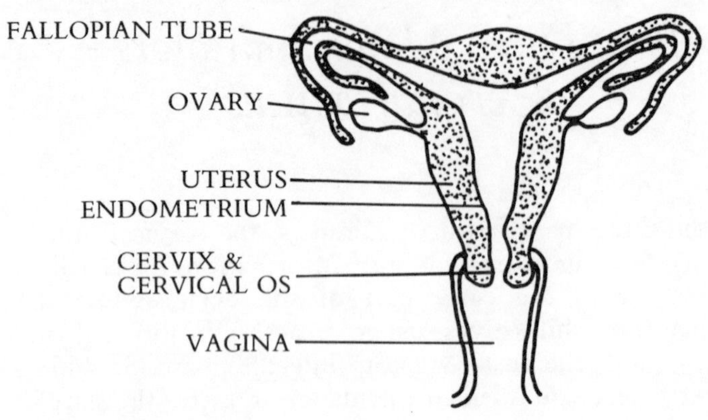

Figure 2. The Woman's Reproductive Anatomy Frontal Cross-Section

In the earliest part of the cycle, immediately after the period, the opening to the cervix, the os, is usually closed with a plug of thick mucus. Therefore no cervical mucus is able to escape into the vagina. The secretions within the vagina are acid and hostile to sperm life – nature's natural spermicide. It is unlikely that spermatazoa can live in this environment for very long, perhaps only a few hours. The sensation at the vaginal entrance, at this stage, is normally one of dryness.

Within a few days, the level of oestrogen still being low, but building up, a small quantity of thick, sticky, whitish even dry and crumbly mucus is produced, which is also inimical to spermatazoa as they cannot swim in this thick mucus. This is known as *less fertile or semi-fertile mucus*. The mucus is produced within the cervix and is brought down slowly by gravity.

Only on the rarest occasions can sperm survive the maximum of five days, some authorities say six to be completely safe, when deposited in this rather unfriendly environment. However, it has happened and so needs to be considered in all calculations of safety (see chapters 7 & 8).

As the cycle progresses with the oestrogen level rising continuously, the mucus becomes thinner and clearer, and a sensation of moistness is experienced. This is the beginning of *fertile mucus*. Then, as the oestrogen level becomes still higher, the mucus becomes more abundant and is positively wet and stretchy like the white of a raw-egg. This mucus is highly *fertile* and indicates imminent ovulation. Fertile mucus nourishes the sperm and allows it to swim through the vagina, cervix and uterus on its journey to meet the ovum. It is often secreted in 'threads', forming channels up which the eager sperm can swim. However, unhealthy sperm of which there are many, are still unable to make the journey and perish either within the vagina or lower down in the cervix. Thus, the mucus has a role in screening only the healthiest sperm to make the long journey through the vagina, into the cervix, along the uterine wall and up the fallopian tube where fertilization will normally take place. In fact, if one examines fertile and infertile mucus under a microscope, one can see very clearly how the former has actual channels within its very watery structure up which the sperm can swim, while infertile mucus is dense and more or less inpenetrable. Having said which, there is evidence that some sperm can occasionally survive acid mucus and can live on for up to five days, within the cervix, as we have mentioned previously.

After ovulation, when the oestrogen level drops off, there is a marked change in the mucus over only a day or two, to the *semi-fertile* and then to the *infertile* pattern. Not infrequently, the change moves directly to the *infertile*. *The last day of fertile mucus,* identified retrospectively, after the return of the dry, semi-fertile or the infertile condition, is known as *Peak Mucus*. Ovulation is thought to occur from two days either side of this day. The rule is:

The post-ovulatory infertile phase begins on the fourth evening past the Peak Mucus or on the third morning of significant temperature shift, WHICHEVER IS THE LATER.

If you are *only* using the mucus indicator, then add an extra day for safety, making it five in all, and see if perhaps there is a return to fertile mucus – which would indicate that it was not *Peak Mucus,* but probably an *attempted* ovulation, with a true ovulation still to come. The four days are calculated as follows: two days for possible ovulation, plus one day for a second ovulation, plus one day for the life of the ovum.

We strongly recommend that the mucus indications always be combined with the detection of a temperature shift. This is because, firstly, the temperature shift is a more positive and objectively identifiable indicator and, secondly, there can be long cycles with more than one patch of fertile mucus, as the level of oestrogen fluctuates according to stress and so on. A cross-checking of peak mucus *and* a temperature shift is a very sure indication that you have reached the post-ovulatory infertile phase.

Note that the *Peak Day* may not be the day of the most abundant mucus, nor the wettest or stretchiest, in fact, there may only have been a residual feeling of wetness. It is identified as being the *last day of fertile mucus*.

During the post-ovulatory infertile phase, as the oestrogen level drops, the mucus remains of the infertile type or there may be none at all. However, just prior to menstruation the cervix may open up to allow the flow and you may get a few days of apparently semi-fertile mucus.

During your period, you will be unable to check the mucus and it is then the cycle starts all over again. But you should start recording mucus on day six, even if there is still some small menstrual flow.

Being Aware of Cervical Mucus

There are really two distinct ways of observing the state of your cervical mucus. Firstly by *visual observation* and secondly by the *sensation* at the vaginal opening, the *labia*. This second method is available even to blind people and is akin to being aware of the different sensations one has of being clean and freshly bathed or of being hot and sweaty after exercise – where visual observation is not required.

Observations of the mucus should be made during the day either as you go about your activities or, particularly, when you go to the bathroom. Then, in the evening, the most fertile condition noted should be recorded. This is the decision you need to make:

Is the mucus condition infertile, semi-fertile or fertile?

Here are some of the key words that will describe the 'standard' circumstances.

INFERTILE	Dry, continuously the same. In 'non-standard' patterns, you may observe flaky, crumbly or thick mucus, sometimes even moist.
SEMI-FERTILE	Flaky, crumbly, thick, moist, milky, tacky, damp, pasty, cloudy, whitish, vinegary, any change from yesterday.★
FERTILE	Wet, stretchy, lubricative, slippery, clear, thin, like egg-white, glossy, transparent, sweet, increased volume, any significant change from yesterday.★

★The importance of *any (significant) change* is given below. It refers mostly to women who have a pattern of continuous mucus, with no totally dry days where mucus is altogether absent.

Basic Infertile Pattern

What you are looking for is:

1. Your *basic infertile pattern.* With most women, this will be dry with no mucus – this is the 'standard' pattern. But with a small percentage, it may be a pattern of continuous dryish and thick, or even moist, mucus. This is the INFERTILE condition, experienced immediately after your period.
2. A *change* towards fertile mucus. This may be any of the descriptions listed under SEMI-FERTILE. If your basic infertile pattern is dry, then *any mucus* of thick, dryish or moist type is SEMI-FERTILE. If you are never dry, then the thick mucus will be INFERTILE, while any change in moisture content will be SEMI-FERTILE.
3. FERTILE mucus is as wet and slippery as it gets with any individual.

You can see, therefore, why it is necessary to observe a full cycle, maybe two, before you start making real assessments as to the mucus type.

Vaginal Sensation

The first way of checking the mucus condition is by how the vaginal entrance *feels*. Does it feel positively dry, even itchy? Is it damp or moist? Or is it wet and slippery? As the days go by, you should be able to note the differences. Note, however, that the vaginal secretions due to sexual excitement and making love, as well as seminal fluid in the vagina, will make the observations difficult and it is useful if you can abstain as much as possible during your learning period, especially at critical times when you are looking for and expecting changes. Normally, when recording regularly, you will not be able to record your mucus for 12 to 24 hours after making love. Double-checking against the cervix itself (see Chapter 6), can be of considerable help here. Most authorities recommend complete abstinence for the first cycle, and while this really is very helpful if you can do it, we wonder how many couples can. One can take it in a positive manner and develop other ways of demonstrating affection, and this would be ideal. But a month . . . ! We certainly recommend waiting until you have recorded a positive temperature shift, indicating that you are in the post-ovulatory infertile phase.

Visual Observation

The cervical mucus can be observed either at the vaginal entrance or from the cervix itself. Using a tissue, you should wipe yourself both before and after urinating, collecting the mucus from the vaginal opening. The mucus collected beforehand would otherwise be washed away, while that collected afterwards has been moved down the vagina by urination. Observe the mucus for the characteristics listed above. The stretchiness can be observed by opening the folds of the tissue with any mucus that stretches more than half an inch being considered as fertile. It will also normally be wet, glistening, transparent and like egg-white and can stretch several inches.

In the 'standard' pattern, semi-fertile mucus is crumbly, thicker, cloudy and not so inclined to stretch into threads, if at all.

Mucus can also be observed on your underwear. We should mention here that cotton is always preferable to nylon or polyester, being a natural fibre. Cotton also absorbs moisture, while man-made fibres may induce a feeling of wetness, quite unrelated to cervical mucus secretions.

Mucus can also be collected from the cervix itself, by inserting your forefinger and index finger into the vagina with one finger tip either side of the cervical opening or os. Applying just a little pressure, bring them together and then, keeping them together, withdraw them and examine the mucus. Opening the two fingers will give you a clear idea of its stretchiness.

Which method you choose is up to you, according to whichever gives you the clearest picture. The advantages of checking the mucus on the cervix itself is that it may otherwise take a day or sometimes more, to travel down to the vaginal entrance. It is thus possible that pregnancy can occur on the last day of a dry vaginal sensation, because although mucus was present on the cervix, it had not yet worked its way down to the vaginal opening. Also, it is a test that can be made in the morning, before you get up, when the vaginal entrance may be dry, and when you want to know your degree of fertility if wondering whether or not to make love. "Milking" the cervix in this way is also unaffected by other vaginal discharges or infections.

You should note that the vagina itself will always be moist or wet – these are different secretions and that is why mucus is observed either at the entrance or on the cervix itself.

Your fingers should, of course, be clean before insertion, but only ordinary washing is necessary, not disinfectant!

When to Observe

You should make the vaginal labia observations during the course of the day whenever you go to the bathroom, but the direct, internal cervical mucus observation should only be done twice a day, say morning and evening, to allow enough time for mucus to accumulate.

Non-Standard Mucus Patterns

Mucus conditions vary from woman to woman more than any of the other natural indicators of fertility. What we have described is the pattern most commonly encountered. In fact, there is a significant number of completely normal women who will have variations on the theme, not only from person to person, but also from cycle to cycle in the same person. This is why it is suggested that you observe your mucus for a couple of cycles before placing any reliance upon this method alone. Don't worry if you can't make the decisions to begin with. Persevere and your own pattern and sensations will become clear to you.

The two extremes of the mucus pattern occur in those women with a continuous sensation of dampness or wetness and those with very little mucus. For these situations, you need to look for *changes* in the mucus, more or less exhibiting a tendency towards the norm. In the case of very little mucus, then vaginal sensation becomes the important indicator since even a little mucus can create a significant feeling. A method recommended by Katia and Jonathan Drake, (Natural Family Planning teachers in London and authors of the book: *Natural Birth Control*) is to contract the muscles around the vagina – the same muscles that are used to stop urinating mid-stream. This contraction and then relaxation helps to bring the cervical mucus down to the vaginal opening. This is a Kegel exercise.

Making Love in the Pre-Ovulatory Infertile Phase

While in the pre-ovulatory infertile phase and watching for the presence of mucus, making love will obscure your observations, because of vaginal secretions and seminal fluid. This is normally cleared within twelve to twenty four hours, but since a day's observation is missed, the rule is:

Dry day, safe night, skip a day

If you are using the cervical condition as an indicator too (see next chapter), then skipping a day will not be necessary if the cervix still indicates the time as infertile.

Disturbances to the Cervical Mucus

As with the temperature indicator, there are a number of environmental and other factors which influence the mucus condition, just as they do the fertility cycle in general. It is, of course, largely related to the hormones controlling the sequence which are themselves the messengers of one's environmental and general physical, emotional and mental input.

Infection may cause a discharge that is irritating, yellow, profuse and even with an unpleasant odour. This will normally make mucus recordings unreliable or impossible. In any event, it is not a good idea to make love when you have any vaginal infection or unusual discharge.

Drugs that include female hormones, tranquillizers, those that dry up mucous membranes (e.g. cold and 'flu drugs), and also cortisones, are known to affect the mucus, making observations unreliable. If in doubt, simply be aware of the possibility and act accordingly. It has been established that insulin does not affect the pattern of cervical mucus, so diabetics can practice these methods with confidence.

Stress, Illness and Emotional Upset can disturb the fertility cycle as we discussed in the previous chapter. What can happen is that as the level of oestrogen fluctuates, so too does the mucus, to such an extent that you may have patches of fertile and patches of infertile mucus changing over. Or you may remain altogether dry. This can be dangerous if you fail to record the possibility of disturbance. These possibilities emphasise why the mucus indicators should be combined with the temperature check to identify, without any doubt, the post-ovulatory phase.

The possibility of an unplanned pregnancy is considerably increased particularly where there is a history of irregular cycles if the mucus indicators are used alone during a time of stress.

Anovulatory cycles too, may be dry or patchy, reflecting nature's struggles towards ovulation.

Using the Cervical Mucus Indicator To Become Pregnant

The cervical mucus method, together with monitoring the cervical condition (Chapter 6) and the Luteinizing Hormone urine dipstick test are the best methods of assessing your times of maximum fertility and for achieving a pregnancy. Basically, you should start making love as soon as the fertile mucus is fully established and hope for the best! If the man has a low, live sperm count and needs to conserve his semen, then you need to pick your time to be as close to *Peak Mucus* as possible. *OVIA,* the fertility assessor described in Chapter 8, has a neat way of predicting this, derived from a calendar calculation, plus a knowledge of past cycles, as well as the current mucus and cervix conditions.

CHAPTER 6

The Three Major Indicators – The Cervix

Checking the condition or state of the cervix itself is really an extension of checking the cervical mucus. Physiologically and anatomically, the cervix changes are part and parcel of the same aspects of the fertility cycle, induced by the changing levels of oestrogen and progesterone. It can be considered as an optional, extra safe-guard and triple-check. If you find it convenient and easy, then it is highly recommended; if you don't want to do it, or you find it unacceptable, then there is no need. However, if you are in doubt about making a sure assessment of your mucus, then the cervix indications may be the answer. If your difficulties are related to low oestrogen levels and anovulatory cycles though, the ambiguity of the mucus may also be reflected in the cervix itself.

Similarly, the cervix becomes a useful indicator when approaching menopause, or at other times when the mucus indicator has been disturbed by the changing hormone levels or other factors.

Finding Your Cervix

Many women have never discovered their cervix and so some preliminary exploration is usually required. There may be some reluctance, pyschologically, to go exploring in those nether regions. However, it is an essential part of your body and worth knowing about. If surgeons and doctor's can poke around and even, under the safety of an anaesthetic, make holes and cut pieces out, surely it must be all right for you to examine yourself privately, in your own home?

Firstly, you need to establish an easy position in which to find the cervix. Because the cervix is at its lowest in the post-ovulatory infertile phase, just before your period, this is a good time for you to start making observations. There are a number of positions which you can check out.

1. Try with one leg up on a chair or the side of the bath.
2. Squatting on your heels with your knees apart.
3. Lying on your back with your knees in the air and legs apart.

It is a good idea to urinate first, because a full bladder can make the cervix high up and difficult to reach. But note that a bowel movement can cause the os to open a little, so do the one, but not the other!

Then, using either your middle finger alone or both your middle and index fingers together, reach up inside and try to find the cervix. It will be centrally located or perhaps a little over to one side. Its surface is smooth, unlike the ridged walls of the vagina, but not as soft. Being cylindrical, you should be able to run the tip of your finger around it and the opening, or os, will be identifiable as a dimple (if closed), or as an opening that can be large enough to admit your finger. The cervix has been described variously as like a narrow chin (with a dimple), like a nose (with a dimple) or like the narrow end of a pear (without the stalk!)

If you have trouble finding it, you can try pressing down gently with the palm of your hand on your lower abdomen. If you still have trouble finding it yourself, you could ask your husband to try, but then you might both get distracted from the original object you had in mind!

When you have decided on the best method for you to identify your cervix, then you should stick to that exactly for at least the complete cycle, because the different postures will put the cervix into different positions and your assessment is based on its relative, day-to-day, positions.

Cervical Changes Throughout the Fertility Cycle

The cervix is the more or less cylindrical lower end of the uterus, about one inch in diameter, projecting downwards from the lower abdomen into the upper end of the vagina.

In the early, relatively infertile phase of your cycle, just after your period has ended, the opening is either closed, or plugged with dry mucus. If you have had a baby, it may never be totally closed.

As the level of oestrogen builds up, so the uterine walls contract and the cervix is drawn up by as much as an inch sometimes even to a point out of reach. Its surface becomes softer, even spongy or rubbery, and you can feel first the tacky or sticky mucus and then the more fertile mucus on its exterior, as the os opens and the fertile mucus is secreted. The os may open up enough to admit the end of your finger, the changes being quite distinct.

Nature's purpose in all this is pretty clear – to make conditions friendly towards sperm and allow the healthiest of them to swim up to meet the ovum.

The changes may be summarized as follows and you should find that they will correlate with the mucus only indicators.

INFERTILE	Firm, dimpled, os closed, surface dry or even gritty.
SEMI-FERTILE	Ripening, rising, softening, sticky or tacky, any change from the infertile state, os opening.
FERTILE	Soft, rubbery, spongy, slippery, os fully open, higher up, any change from the semi-fertile state.

Ovulation occurs more or less synchronously with the peak of the fertile condition and then, with the rise in the level of progesterone, the cervix reverts quite rapidly to its infertile state. The cervix closes off, the uterus relaxes with a subsequent fall in the cervical position and the mucus once again becomes thick and hostile to sperm, or there is no mucus at all.

Towards the end of the cycle, the os opens up to allow the menstrual flow and then closes again, immediately the period is over.

When to Observe the Cervix

We recommend that you start checking the cervix during the post-ovulatory, infertile phase of your cycle, when it is at its lowest point and the most easily felt. Then, starting again after your period, but not later than day six, even if there is still some minor blood spotting, you can observe a full cycle of cervical events. After two or three cycles, you should be conversant enough with the changes to incorporate them into your chosen method of fertility assessment, though some women do take up to six months to be totally sure of their cervix indications.

Check your cervix not more than once or twice a day, since it may interfere with the mucus observations, the best times being midday and evening, or just in the evening. As with the mucus, always record the most fertile condition. Since the cervix position can vary during the course of a day, it can be preferable to check it just in the evening only. The cervix is generally higher up in the morning than in the evening.

The Infertility Rule

The rule, for maximum safety against conception, is:

The first safe day in the post-ovulatory infertile phase is four full days after you have observed the return to the infertile cervical state.

As always, we recommend the cross-checking of all three indicators. For your fertility assessment in the other phases of the cycle, see Chapters 7 and 8.

Variations and Disturbances

As with the mucus signs, there may be variations from woman to woman and cycle to cycle, but they are not vastly different and the cervix signs can be used as a cross-check whenever the mucus indicators are unclear. The principle of *change* still applies, however, in cases where it is difficult to notice the other factors.

The effects of emotional upset and stress on the hormones levels will also be reflected in the cervical state, as with the other indicators, and you need to take note of such possible disturbances. Childbirth, too, will change your cervical condition and it may take a while to settle down again, (see Chapter 10). The basic infertile state of the cervical opening will almost certainly be incompletely closed after your first child, though it may have been totally closed beforehand. During the infertile phases, the os remains plugged with thick, dry mucus. Sometimes, due to cervical *erosions* – when the interior lining of the cervix grows out over the exterior – there can be an unusually large discharge of mucus. This can be medically dealt with if it is a nuisance or uncomfortable and there are herbal and natural remedies, too. Finally, any operation on the cervix – cervical cancer for example – normally removes a part of it, including the mucus producing tissues, which will clearly alter your observations.

Reliability

Cervical indices of fertility are comparatively new and although well researched and correlated with the other indicators, no long-term statistical study has yet been undertaken. Dr. Anna Flynn's current research at the Birmingham Maternity Hospital is definitely revealing the cervix as a major, highly reliable indicator. Our own feeling is that the next major study should cover women using all the available indicators. The new *OVIA* fertility assessor should be able to provide a considerable amount of statistical data on the use of the combined indicators from questionnaires distributed to its users.

CHAPTER 7

Fertility Assessment – Using a Chart

Having covered all the well researched and readily recordable indices of fertility, we now need to put this information together in the easiest ways possible in order to make an accurate assessment of fertility. There are currently only two reliable ways of doing this.

1. Either you can use a specially worked out chart and make your assessment according to the rules and indications given throughout this book and summarized in this chapter, or
2. You can use the electronic fertility assesser, *OVIA*, upon which you record your data and which accurately, immediately and objectively, makes the assessment for you.

In this chapter, we explain how to use a chart for assessing your degree of fertility, so first of all, please examine the blank Chart 1. It is essential that the chart be well-designed so that it is simple to read and interpret. Temperatures must be spaced at 0.05°C/0.1°F in square boxes and all the other details must be well laid out.

Charting Your Period

Day 1 of your cycle is by convention taken as the first day of your period. This should be entered a a 'P' in the relevant row on the chart for each day of your period.

Charting Your Temperature

*Complete the chart each morning by putting a dot in the centre of the relevant square and joining it up to the previous day.

★Make any adjustments for late or early rising (if you are confident of the degree of adjustment) before you record the temperature, otherwise put a cross in the "disturbed" row and record the temperature just as you took it.

★Mark any suspected disturbances in the "disturbed" row. This includes illness, a cold, a long journey, emotional upset, etc.

Remember that the temperature shift is to enable you to predict the start of the post-ovulatory infertile phase. The rule is:

The post-ovulatory infertile phase begins on the third morning of a sustained temperature shift greater than or equal to 0.2°C/ 0.4°F, all three of which are greater than any of the temperatures taken on the previous six days; or the fourth evening after the last day of fertile mucus (Peak Mucus); or fertile cervix signs, WHICHEVER IS THE LATER.

The easiest way to detect this temperature rise is to draw a *cover line* above the six lower temperatures and below the three higher temperatures. You can also, if you wish, draw a *shift line* on the day of the first higher temperature, to pinpoint the probable day of ovulation.

Chart 2 shows the classical pattern of a mid-cycle temperature rise with the cover and shift lines drawn in. Many women find that their temperature rise follows this classical pattern, month after month. However, one does need to be aware of variations, best exemplified by studying charts 2–10, while reading through the followed notes, ignoring the mucus and cervix annotations for the moment.

Chart 3 shows three temperature spikes, one in the early pre-ovulatory phase, one in the six days prior to the temperature shift and one in the post-ovulatory infertile phase. These could be due to any of the normal causes of disturbed readings, including a sore throat or a cold, but certainly not 'flu. All of them may be safely ignored.

Chart 4 shows a temperature rise due to 'flu in the early phase and then a temperature spike right at the start of the three higher temperatures. This day was marked as being potentially disturbed and is therefore *not counted* as one of the three higher temperatures. The rule is:

The three higher temperatures must not include any suspect or disturbed temperatures. Keep counting until you have three reliable, consecutive higher temperatures.

If you have 'flu mid-cycle, then you need to wait until you are sure that all the temperature symptoms have gone before looking for three temperatures, higher than six *before* you got 'flu. And don't forget that illness may in any case have delayed ovulation, so don't be over anxious to find the temperature shift and make a mistake.

Chart 5 shows how the temperature rise can be irregular during a cycle and may also rise in a step-like fashion. In this case, always wait until the situation has clarified itself, delaying a few extra days until you are sure. All pre-ovulatory days are marked as potentially fertile on this chart, because we are not recording mucus or cervical indicators.

Chart 6 shows how the temperature rise can, occasionally, be in the nature of a saw-tooth. Here, the three over six rule does not work and yet the temperature rise is still apparent. The rule here is:

Wait until the situation has clarified itself before assuming that you are infertile.

You need to be sure that the basic pattern of temperature is the normal 0.2°C/0.4°F above the pre-ovulatory temperatures.

Chart 7 shows a very short cycle.

Chart 8 shows a very long one.

Chart 9 shows how an *anovulatory cycle,* often long, rambles on and on, never quite making an ovulation. Perhaps the oestrogen level is fluctuating as the body tries to reach a state where ovulation would be possible. Perhaps stress is keeping the level at a point where ovulation cannot occur – nature's way of avoiding a pregnancy in a situation where the potential mother is already under enough stress and may not be able to cope with being pregnant. In this instance, from the temperature alone one can determine very little concerning fertility, except that ovulation has not occurred.

Chart 10 shows a probable pregnancy. The temperature rise is sustained for more than twenty days and the dates of making love recorded. From our knowledge of when ovulation occurred, we can calculate the date of birth as:

Date of temperature shift minus 7 plus 9 calendar months

It is great fun to be able to confirm your doctor's prognosis and show him exactly how you knew!

Charting Your Mucus

You should begin observing and recording your mucus only after your period has ended. There have been a number of ways devised for charting your mucus, some more complex than others, some using symbols and some colours. The problem with symbols and colours is remembering what they are or what they mean, while letters can be ambiguous. 'I', for example, may stand for 'Infertile' or 'Intercourse', while 'M' can stand for 'Moist' or 'Mucus'. 'D' can stand for 'Dry', which is also 'Infertile'. Most women have 'Dry' days, taken to be the infertile days, and then move on to what is variously called 'infertile mucus' or 'less-fertile mucus' and finally 'Wet' or 'fertile mucus'. Other women have no 'Dry' days but a mucus which they come to recognise as their 'Infertile mucus', with a certain difference in its condition characterised as their 'less-fertile mucus', any further changes being recognised as their 'fertile mucus'.

It is for these reasons that a good chart will always have two rows for entering your mucus record. One will hold a key to your mucus and its type, while the other will allow you to describe its nature in your own words. This is very helpful while learning in the early days, to allow you to compare, in retrospect, one day with another and one cycle with another.

Because of this confusion, and after considerable deliberation, we have decided to introduce yet another variation on the theme. We think that our system does provide some clarification, but we certainly don't deny the advantages of other ways of doing it, particularly if you

Natural Fertility Awareness

Chart No: ______ Year: ______

Usual time of taking temperature ______

Last 6–12 cycles { Shortest: ______ Longest: ______

This cycle length: ______

Shortest Cycle – 20 ______

Minor Indicators

O Ovulation pain
S Blood spotting
B Breasts tender or sore
F Feeling of fullness/heaviness
E Emotional upset

Temperature Rise in Previous Cycle: YES/NO

Name: ....

Date									
37.25	99.3								
37.20	99.2								
37.15	99.1								
37.10	99.0								
37.05	98.9								
37.00	98.8								
36.95	98.7								
36.90	98.6								
36.85	98.5								
36.80	98.4								
36.75	98.3								
36.70	98.2								
36.65	98.1								
36.60	98.0								
36.55	97.9								
36.50	97.8								
36.45	97.7								
36.40	97.6								
36.35	97.5								
36.30	97.4								
36.25	97.3								
36.20	97.2								
36.15	97.1								
36.10	97.0								
36.05	96.9								
36.00	96.8								
Day		1	2	3	4	5	6	7	8

	Code	1	2	3	4	5	6	7	8
Period	P								
Mucus I Infertile S Semi Fertile F Fertile Ⓕ Peak Mucus	I S F Ⓕ Verbal Description								
Cervix f firm s soft	f s ● ● ● ○ ○ ○ I S F								
Minor Indicators	O S B F E								
Disturbed/ill	D								
Made Love/Sexual Contact	L								
Fertility Assessment	X/								

Chart 1 – Blank Chart

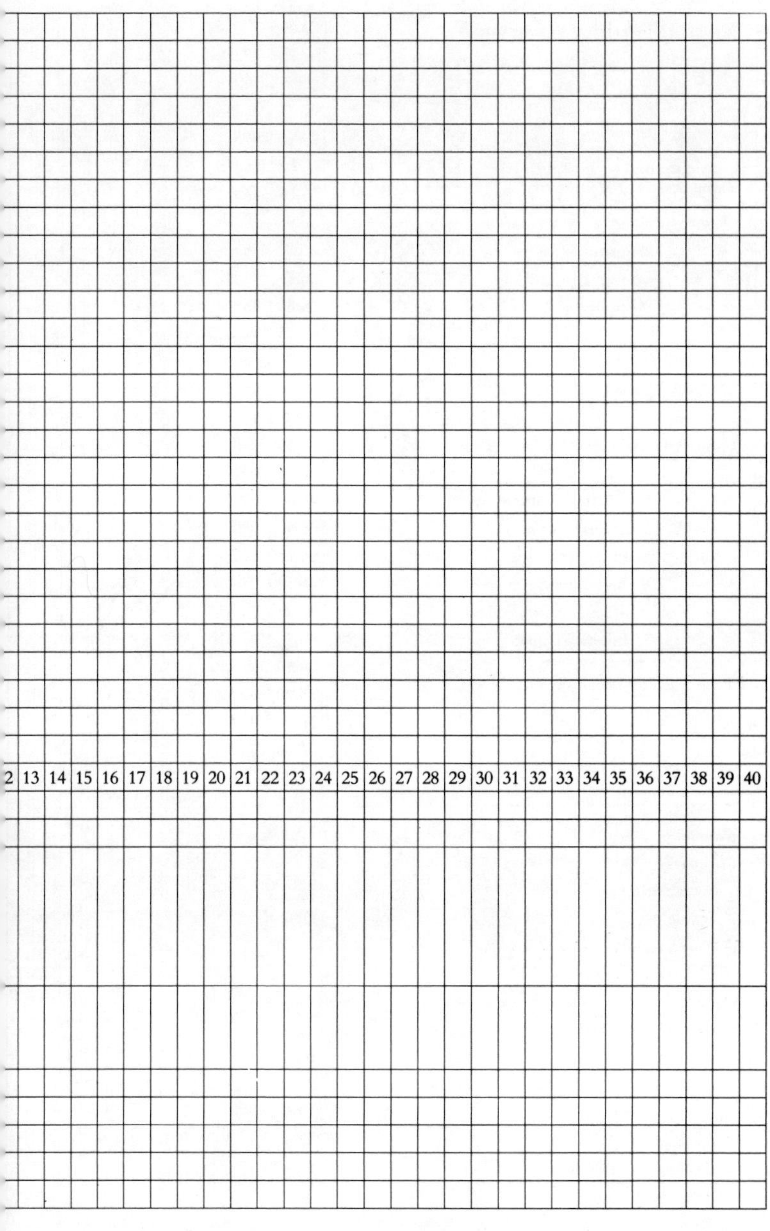
2 13 14 15 16 17 18 19 20 21 22 23 24 25 26 27 28 29 30 31 32 33 34 35 36 37 38 39 40

Natural Fertility Awareness

Chart No: [ ] Year: [ ]

Usual time of taking temperature [ ]

Last 6–12 cycles { Shortest: 28 / Longest: 28 }

This cycle length: 28

Shortest Cycle – 20: 8

Minor Indicators

- O Ovulation pain
- S Blood spotting
- B Breasts tender or sore
- F Feeling of fullness/heaviness
- E Emotional upset

Temperature Rise in Previous Cycle: (YES) NO

Name: ....

Date									
37.25	99.3								
37.20	99.2								
37.15	99.1								
37.10	99.0								
37.05	98.9								
37.00	98.8								
36.95	98.7								
36.90	98.6								
36.85	98.5								
36.80	98.4								
36.75	98.3								
36.70	98.2								
36.65	98.1								
36.60	98.0								
36.55	97.9								
36.50	97.8								
36.45	97.7								
36.40	97.6								
36.35	97.5								
36.30	97.4								
36.25	97.3								
36.20	97.2								
36.15	97.1								
36.10	97.0								
36.05	96.9								
36.00	96.8								

	Code	1	2	3	4	5	6	7	8
	Day	1	2	3	4	5	6	7	8
Period	P	P	P	P	P	P			
Mucus I Infertile S Semi Fertile F Fertile Ⓕ Peak Mucus	I S F Ⓕ						I	I	I
	Verbal Description						Dry	Dry	Dry
Cervix f firm s soft	f s						f	f	f
	●●●○○○						●	●	●
	I S F						I	I	I
Minor Indicators	O S B F E								
Disturbed/ill	D								
Made Love/Sexual Contact	L								
Fertility Assessment	X/								X

Chart 2 – Normal Patterns of Temperature, Mucus and Cervix

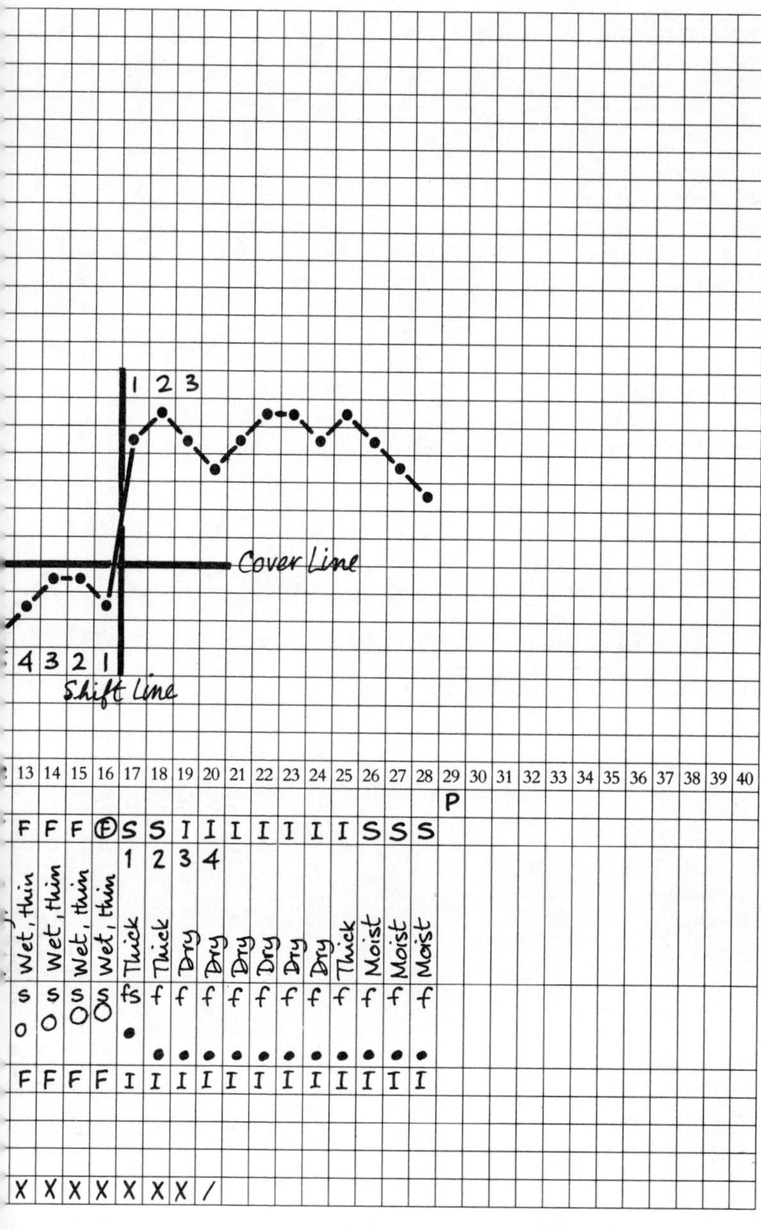
1 2 3
Cover Line
4 3 2 1
Shift Line
13 14 15 16 17 18 19 20 21 22 23 24 25 26 27 28 29 30 31 32 33 34 35 36 37 38 39 40
P
F F F F S S I I I I I I I S S S
1 2 3 4
Wet, thin
Wet, thin
Wet, thin
Wet, thin
Thick
Thick
Dry
Dry
Dry
Dry
Dry
Dry
Thick
Moist
Moist
Moist
s s s s fs f f f f f f f f f f f
o O O On
F F F F I I I I I I I I I I I I
X X X X X X X /

Natural Fertility Awareness

Chart No: [ ] Year: [ ]

Usual time of taking temperature [ ]

Last 6–12 cycles { Shortest: 28 ; Longest: 28 }

This cycle length: 28

Shortest Cycle – 20: 8

Minor Indicators

- O Ovulation pain
- S Blood spotting
- B Breasts tender or sore
- F Feeling of fullness/heaviness
- E Emotional upset

Temperature Rise in Previous Cycle: (YES)/NO

Name: ....

Date									
37.25	99.3								
37.20	99.2								
37.15	99.1								
37.10	99.0								
37.05	98.9								
37.00	98.8								
36.95	98.7								
36.90	98.6								
36.85	98.5								
36.80	98.4								
36.75	98.3								
36.70	98.2								
36.65	98.1								
36.60	98.0						Went to a party		
36.55	97.9								
36.50	97.8						•		
36.45	97.7								
36.40	97.6	•							
36.35	97.5								
36.30	97.4		•		•			•	
36.25	97.3			•					•
36.20	97.2					•			
36.15	97.1								
36.10	97.0								
36.05	96.9								
36.00	96.8								

	Code	1	2	3	4	5	6	7	8
	Day	1	2	3	4	5	6	7	8
Period	P	P	P	P	P	P			
Mucus I Infertile, S Semi Fertile, F Fertile, Ⓕ Peak Mucus	I S F Ⓕ						I	I	I
	Verbal Description						white, thick moist	white, thick moist	white, thick moist
Cervix f firm, s soft	f s						f	f	f
	●●●○○○						●	●	●
	I S F						I	I	I
Minor Indicators	O S B F E								
Disturbed/ill	D						D		
Made Love/Sexual Contact	L								
Fertility Assessment	X/								X

Chart 3 – Normal Patterns with Some Disturbances

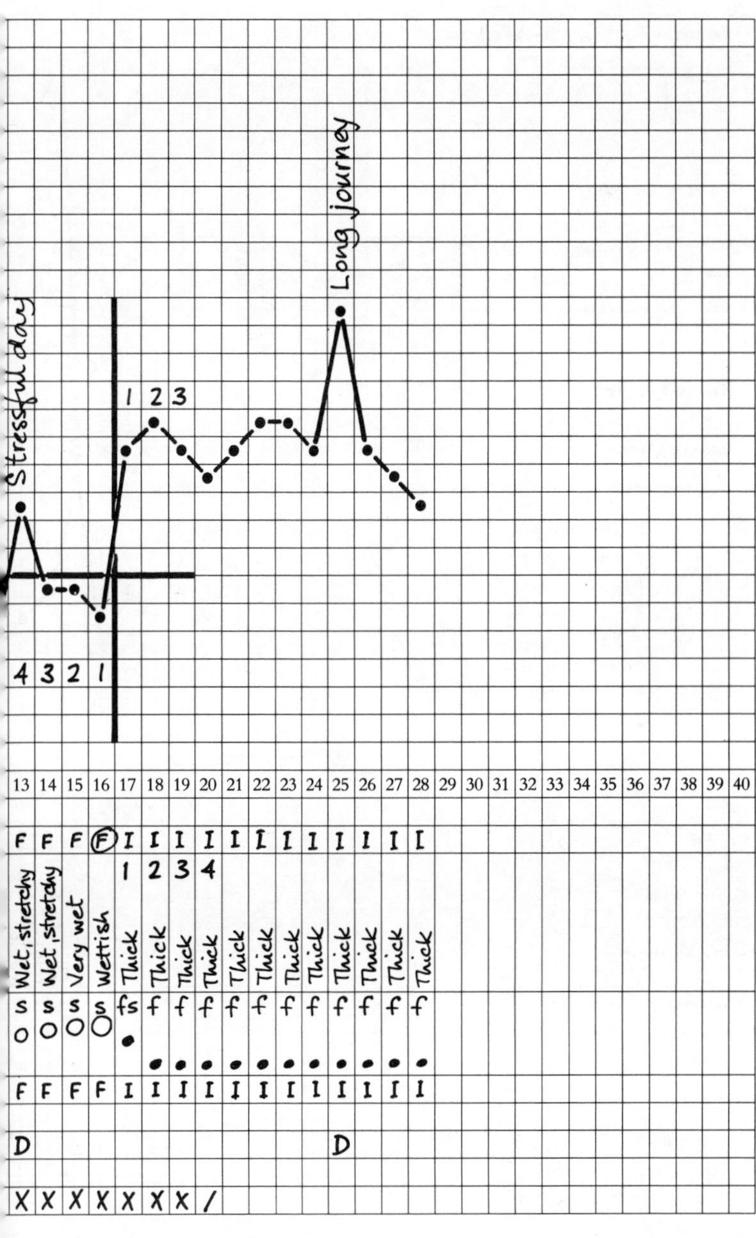
Stressful day
Long journey
1 2 3
4 3 2 1
13 14 15 16 17 18 19 20 21 22 23 24 25 26 27 28 29 30 31 32 33 34 35 36 37 38 39 40
F F F F I I I I I I I I I I I I
1 2 3 4
Wet, stretchy
Wet, stretchy
Very wet
Wettish
Thick
Thick
Thick
Thick
Thick
Thick
Thick
Thick
Thick
Thick
Thick
Thick
s s s s fs f f f f f f f f f f f
F F F F I I I I I I I I I I I I
D
D
X X X X X X X /

Natural Fertility Awareness

Chart No: [ ] Year: [ ]

Usual time of taking temperature [ ]

Last 6–12 cycles — Shortest: 28 — Longest: 28

This cycle length: 28

Shortest Cycle – 20: 8

Minor Indicators

- O Ovulation pain
- S Blood spotting
- B Breasts tender or sore
- F Feeling of fullness/heaviness
- E Emotional upset

Temperature Rise in Previous Cycle: (YES)/NO

Name: ....

Date		1	2	3	4	5	6	7
37.25	99.3							
37.20	99.2							
37.15	99.1							
37.10	99.0							
37.05	98.9							Flu.
37.00	98.8							
36.95	98.7							
36.90	98.6							
36.85	98.5							
36.80	98.4							
36.75	98.3							
36.70	98.2							
36.65	98.1							
36.60	98.0							
36.55	97.9							
36.50	97.8							
36.45	97.7							
36.40	97.6							
36.35	97.5							
36.30	97.4							
36.25	97.3							
36.20	97.2							
36.15	97.1							
36.10	97.0							
36.05	96.9							
36.00	96.8							

	Code	1	2	3	4	5	6	7
Period	P	P	P	P	P	P		
Mucus I Infertile, S Semi Fertile, F Fertile, Ⓕ Peak Mucus	I S F Ⓕ						I	
	Verbal Description						Dry	
Cervix f firm, s soft	f s						f	f
	●●●○○○						●	●
	I S F						I	
Minor Indicators	O S B F E							
Disturbed/ill	D						D	D
Made Love/Sexual Contact	L						L	L
Fertility Assessment	X/							

Chart 4 – Normal Patterns with 'Flu and a Disturbance During a Temperature Shift

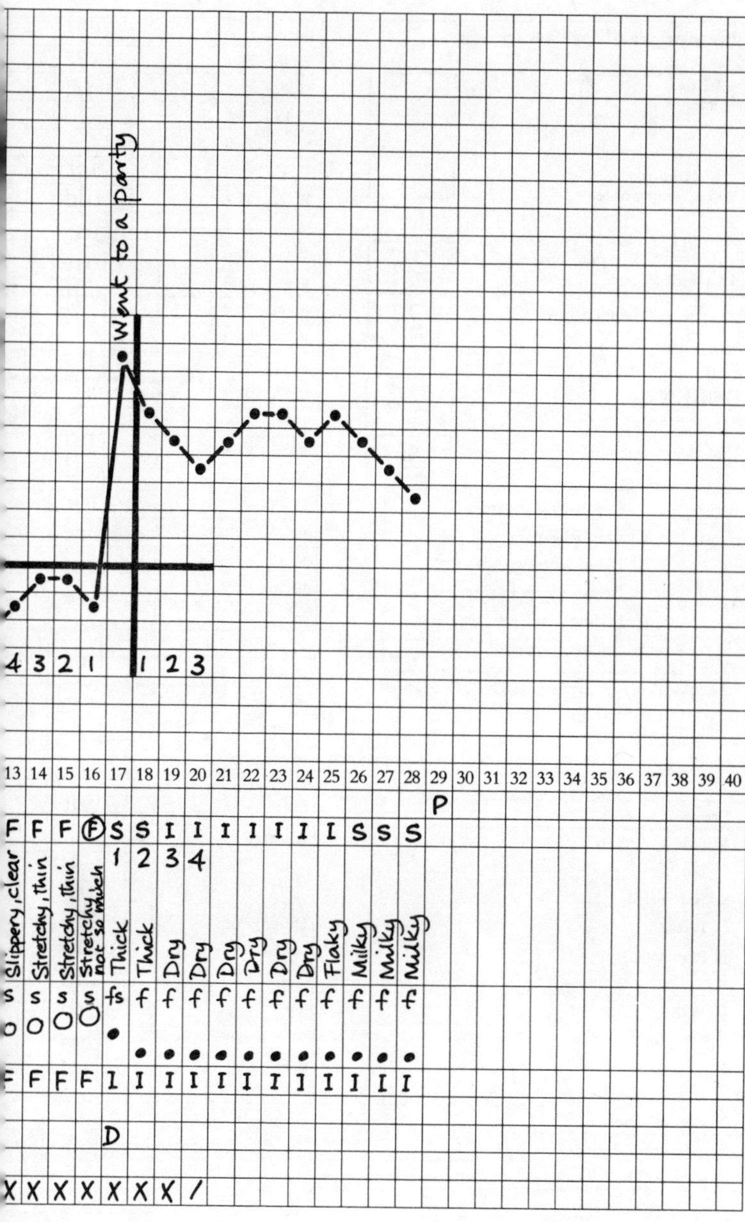
Went to a party
4 3 2 1 1 2 3
13 14 15 16 17 18 19 20 21 22 23 24 25 26 27 28 29 30 31 32 33 34 35 36 37 38 39 40
P
F F F F S S I I I I I I I S S S
1 2 3 4
Slippery, clear
Stretchy, thin
Stretchy, thin
Stretchy not so much
Thick
Thick
Dry
Dry
Dry
Dry
Dry
Dry
Flaky
Milky
Milky
Milky
s s s s fs f f f f f f f f f f f
o O O O
F F F F I I I I I I I I I I I I
D
X X X X X X X /

Natural Fertility Awareness

Chart No: [ ] Year: [ ]

Usual time of taking temperature [ ]

Last 6–12 cycles { Shortest: 28 / Longest: 28 }

This cycle length: 28

Shortest Cycle – 20: 8

Minor Indicators

- O Ovulation pain
- S Blood spotting
- B Breasts tender or sore
- F Feeling of fullness/heaviness
- E Emotional upset

Temperature Rise in Previous Cycle: (YES) NO

Name: ....

Date								
37.25	99.3							
37.20	99.2							
37.15	99.1							
37.10	99.0							
37.05	98.9							
37.00	98.8							
36.95	98.7							
36.90	98.6							
36.85	98.5							
36.80	98.4							
36.75	98.3							
36.70	98.2							
36.65	98.1							
36.60	98.0							
36.55	97.9							
36.50	97.8							6
36.45	97.7							
36.40	97.6							
36.35	97.5							
36.30	97.4							
36.25	97.3							
36.20	97.2							
36.15	97.1							
36.10	97.0							
36.05	96.9							
36.00	96.8							
Code	Day	1	2	3	4	5	6	7
Period	P	P	P	P	P	P		
Mucus I Infertile, S Semi Fertile, F Fertile, Ⓕ Peak Mucus	I S F Ⓕ / Verbal Description							
Cervix f firm, s soft	f s / ●●●○○○ / I S F							
Minor Indicators	O S B F E							
Disturbed/ill	D							
Made Love/Sexual Contact	L							
Fertility Assessment	X/						X	X

Chart 5 – A Step-Like Temperature Rise

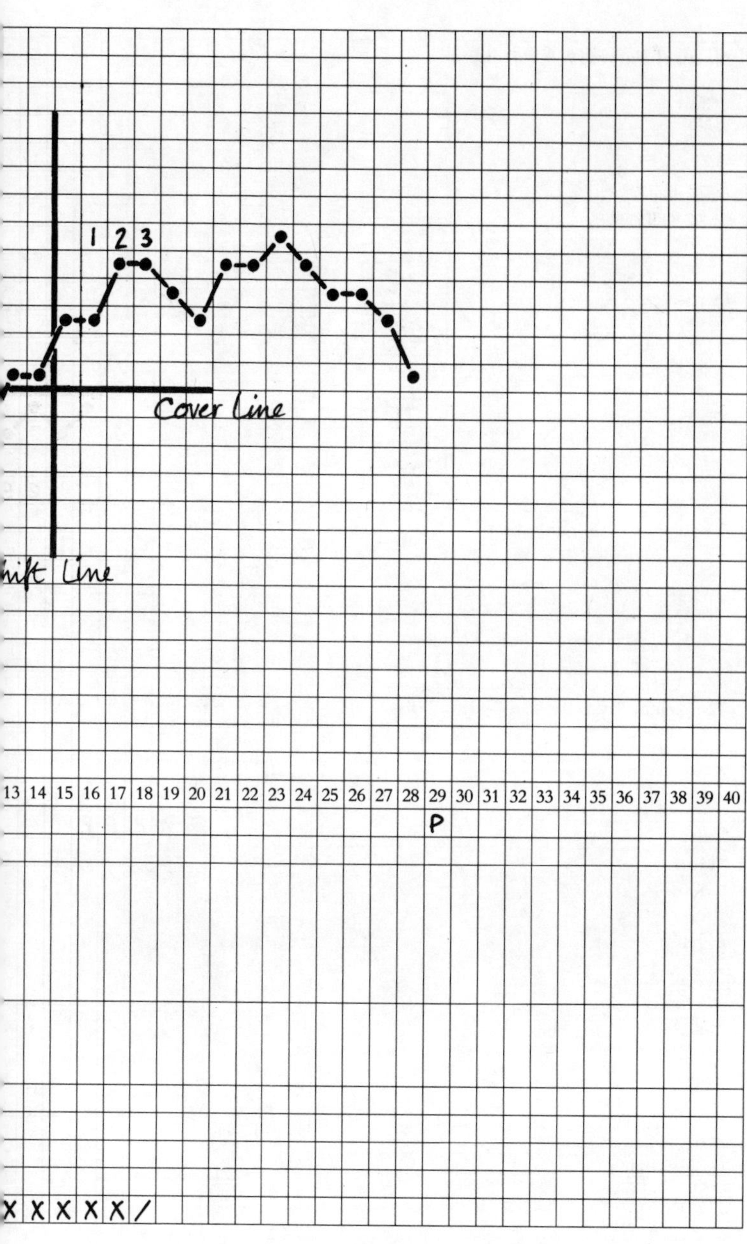
1 2 3
Cover Line
hift Line
13 14 15 16 17 18 19 20 21 22 23 24 25 26 27 28 29 30 31 32 33 34 35 36 37 38 39 40
P
X X X X X /

Natural Fertility Awareness

Chart No: [ ] Year: [ ]

Usual time of taking temperature [ ]

Last 6–12 cycles — Shortest: 28 — Longest: 28

This cycle length: 28

Shortest Cycle – 20: 8

Minor Indicators

- O Ovulation pain
- S Blood spotting
- B Breasts tender or sore
- F Feeling of fullness/heaviness
- E Emotional upset

Temperature Rise in Previous Cycle: (YES) NO

Name: ....

Date									
37.25	99.3								
37.20	99.2								
37.15	99.1								
37.10	99.0								
37.05	98.9								
37.00	98.8								
36.95	98.7								
36.90	98.6								
36.85	98.5								
36.80	98.4								
36.75	98.3								
36.70	98.2								
36.65	98.1								
36.60	98.0								
36.55	97.9								
36.50	97.8								
36.45	97.7								
36.40	97.6								
36.35	97.5								
36.30	97.4								
36.25	97.3								
36.20	97.2								
36.15	97.1								
36.10	97.0								
36.05	96.9								
36.00	96.8								

	Code	Day 1	2	3	4	5	6	7
Period	P	P	P	P	P	P		
Mucus I Infertile S Semi Fertile F Fertile Ⓕ Peak Mucus	I S F Ⓕ						I	I
	Verbal Description						Dry	Dry
Cervix f firm s soft	f s						f	f
	●●●○○○						●	●
	I S F						I	I
Minor Indicators	O S B F E							
Disturbed/ill	D							
Made Love/Sexual Contact	L							
Fertility Assessment	X/							

Chart 6 – A Saw-Tooth Temperature Rise, Clarified by Mucus Indicators

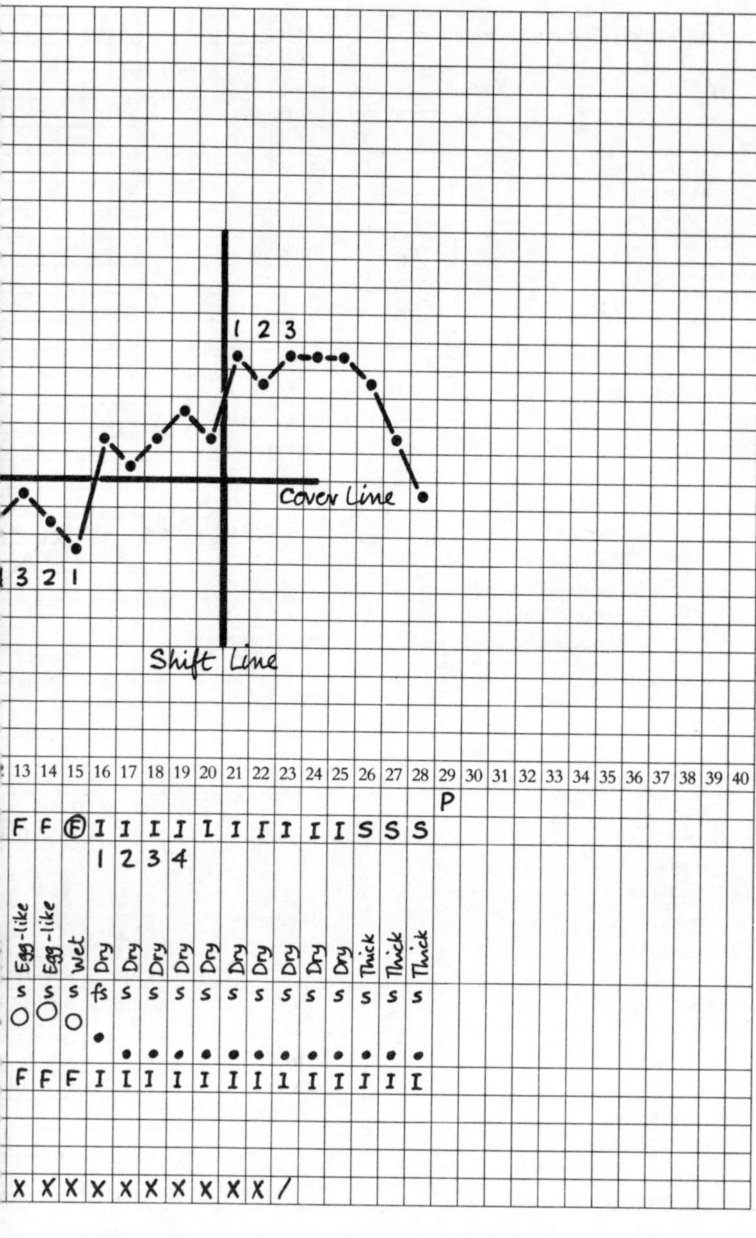

1 2 3
Cover Line
3 2 1
Shift Line
13 14 15 16 17 18 19 20 21 22 23 24 25 26 27 28 29 30 31 32 33 34 35 36 37 38 39 40
P
F F Ⓕ I I I I I I I I I I S S S
1 2 3 4
Egg-like Egg-like Wet Dry Dry Dry Dry Dry Dry Dry Dry Dry Dry Thick Thick Thick
s s s fs s s s s s s s s s s s s
F F F I I I I I I I I I I I I I
X X X X X X X X X X /

Natural Fertility Awareness

Chart No: | Year:

Usual time of taking temperature

Last 6–12 cycles — Shortest: 21 — Longest: 28

This cycle length: 21

Shortest Cycle – 20: 1

Minor Indicators
- O Ovulation pain
- S Blood spotting
- B Breasts tender or sore
- F Feeling of fullness/heaviness
- E Emotional upset

Temperature Rise in Previous Cycle: (YES) / NO

Name: ....

Date	
37.25	99.3
37.20	99.2
37.15	99.1
37.10	99.0
37.05	98.9
37.00	98.8
36.95	98.7
36.90	98.6
36.85	98.5
36.80	98.4
36.75	98.3
36.70	98.2
36.65	98.1
36.60	98.0
36.55	97.9
36.50	97.8
36.45	97.7
36.40	97.6
36.35	97.5
36.30	97.4
36.25	97.3
36.20	97.2
36.15	97.1
36.10	97.0
36.05	96.9
36.00	96.8

Shift

	Code	1	2	3	4	5	6	7	8
	Day	1	2	3	4	5	6	7	8
Period	P	P	P	P					
Mucus	I S F Ⓕ				S	F	F	F	Ⓕ
I Infertile; S Semi Fertile; F Fertile; Ⓕ Peak Mucus	Verbal Description				Thick	Moist	Wet, Slippery	Thin, Stretchy	Thin, Stretchy
Cervix f firm, s soft	f s				fs	s	s	s	s
	●●●○○○	●	●	●	●	o	O	O	O
	I S F				S	F	F	F	F
Minor Indicators	O S B F E								
Disturbed/ill	D								
Made Love/Sexual Contact	L								
Fertility Assessment	X/	X	X	X	X	X	X	X	X

Chart 7 – A Very Short Cycle

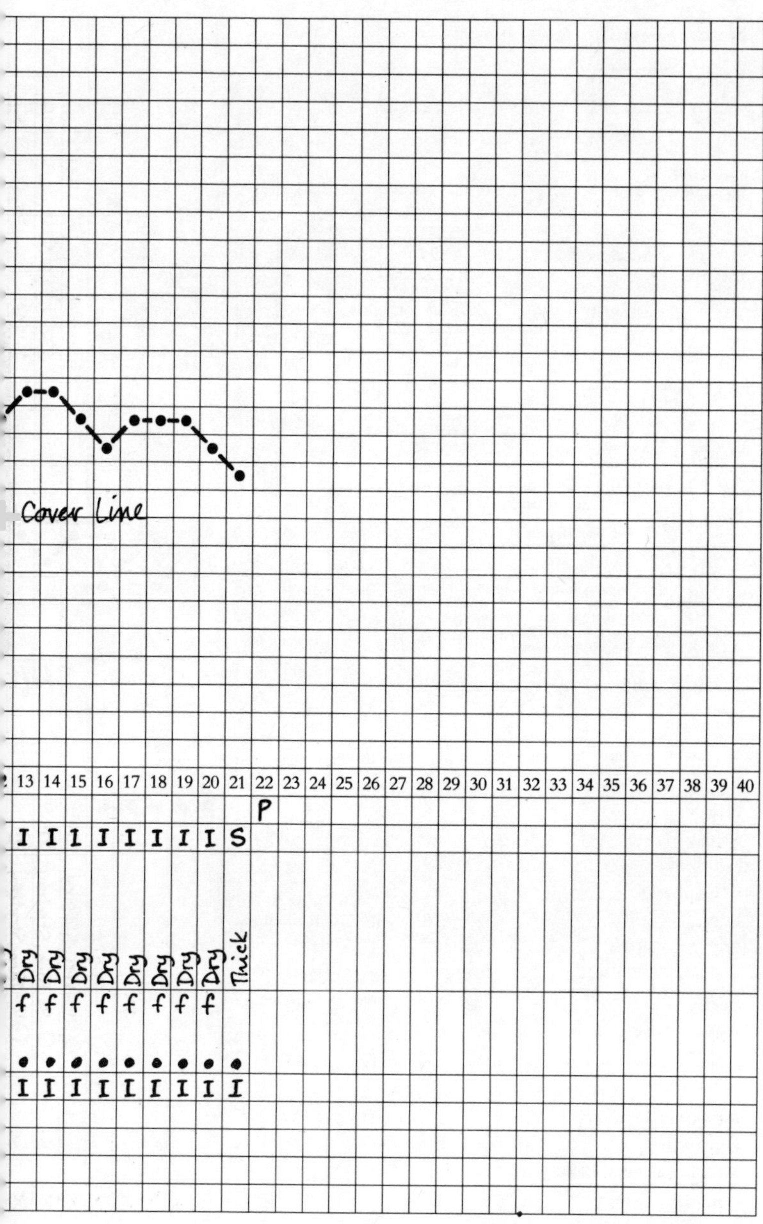

Cover Line
13 14 15 16 17 18 19 20 21 22 23 24 25 26 27 28 29 30 31 32 33 34 35 36 37 38 39 40
P
I I I I I I I I S
Dry Dry Dry Dry Dry Dry Dry Dry Thick
f f f f f f f f
I I I I I I I I I

Natural Fertility Awareness

Chart No: [ ]   Year: [ ]

Usual time of taking temperature [ ]

Last 6–12 cycles — Shortest: 28 — Longest: 40

This cycle length: 39

Shortest Cycle – 20: 8

Minor Indicators

- O Ovulation pain
- S Blood spotting
- B Breasts tender or sore
- F Feeling of fullness/heaviness
- E Emotional upset

Temperature Rise in Previous Cycle: (YES)/NO

Name: ....

Date									
37.25	99.3								
37.20	99.2								
37.15	99.1								
37.10	99.0								
37.05	98.9								
37.00	98.8								
36.95	98.7								
36.90	98.6								
36.85	98.5								
36.80	98.4								
36.75	98.3								
36.70	98.2								
36.65	98.1								
36.60	98.0								
36.55	97.9								
36.50	97.8								
36.45	97.7								
36.40	97.6								
36.35	97.5								
36.30	97.4								
36.25	97.3								
36.20	97.2								
36.15	97.1								
36.10	97.0								
36.05	96.9								
36.00	96.8								

Family crisis requiring late nights and a long journey. Possible cause of ...

	Code	1	2	3	4	5	6	7	8
Period	P	P	P	P	P	P			
Mucus I Infertile, S Semi Fertile, F Fertile, Ⓕ Peak Mucus	I S F Ⓕ						I	I	I
	Verbal Description						Dry	Dry	Dry
Cervix f firm, s soft	f s						f	f	f
	●●●○○○						●	●	●
	I S F						I	I	I
Minor Indicators	O S B F E								
Disturbed/ill	D						D	D	D
Made Love/Sexual Contact	L								
Fertility Assessment	X/								X

Chart 8 – A Very Long Cycle, Perhaps Due to Stress

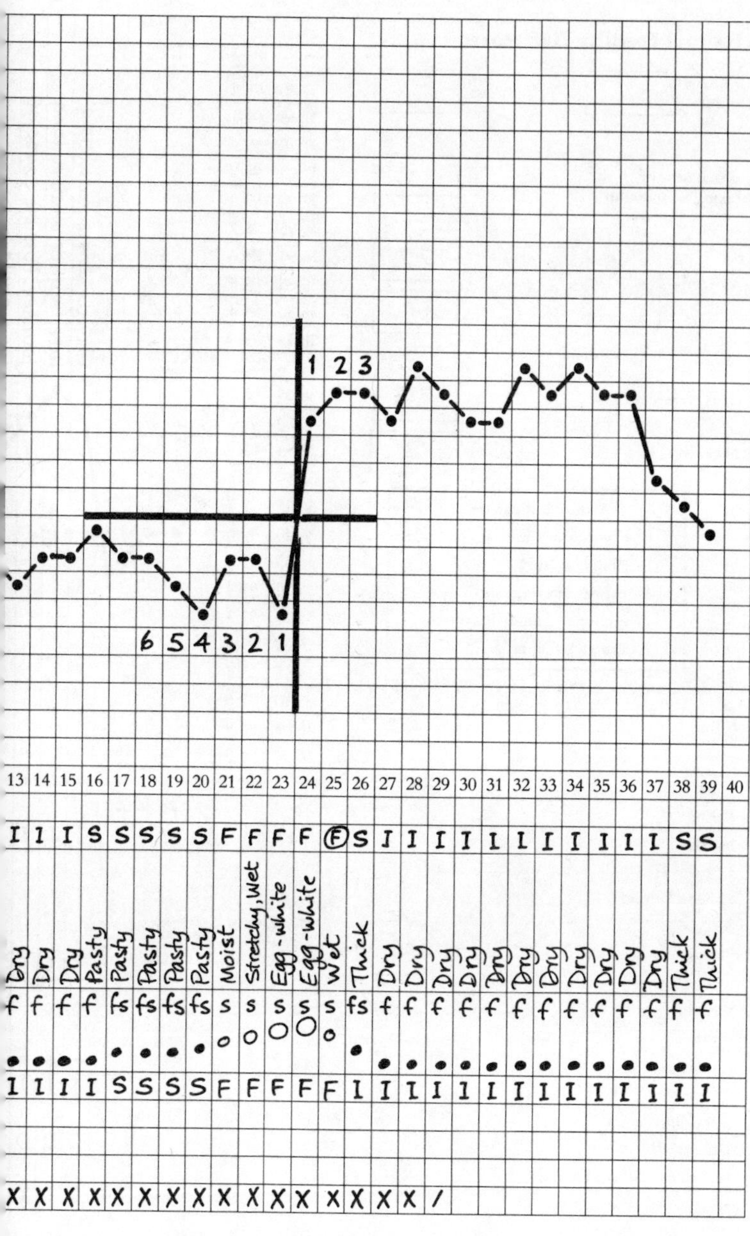
1 2 3
6 5 4 3 2 1
13 14 15 16 17 18 19 20 21 22 23 24 25 26 27 28 29 30 31 32 33 34 35 36 37 38 39 40
I I I S S S S S F F F F Ⓕ S I I I I I I I I I I I S S
Dry Dry Dry Pasty Pasty Pasty Pasty Pasty Moist Stretchy, Wet Egg-white Egg-white Wet Thick Dry Dry Dry Dry Dry Dry Dry Dry Dry Dry Dry Thick Thick
f f f f fs fs fs fs s s s s s fs f f f f f f f f f f f f f
I I I I S S S S F F F F F I I I I I I I I I I I I I I
X X X X X X X X X X X X X X X X /

Natural Fertility Awareness

Chart No: [ ] Year: [ ]

Usual time of taking temperature [ ]

Last 6–12 cycles { Shortest: 22 / Longest: 45

This cycle length: 39

Shortest Cycle – 20: 2

Minor Indicators
- O Ovulation pain
- S Blood spotting
- B Breasts tender or sore
- F Feeling of fullness/heaviness
- E Emotional upset

Temperature Rise in Previous Cycle: YES/NO (NO circled)

Name: ....

Date									
37.25	99.3								
37.20	99.2								
37.15	99.1								
37.10	99.0								
37.05	98.9								
37.00	98.8								
36.95	98.7								
36.90	98.6								
36.85	98.5								
36.80	98.4								
36.75	98.3								
36.70	98.2								
36.65	98.1								
36.60	98.0								•
36.55	97.9								
36.50	97.8								
36.45	97.7	•						•	
36.40	97.6		•	•		•	•		
36.35	97.5				•				
36.30	97.4								
36.25	97.3								
36.20	97.2								
36.15	97.1								
36.10	97.0								
36.05	96.9								
36.00	96.8								
Code	Day	1	2	3	4	5	6	7	8
Period	P	P	P	P	P	P			
Mucus	I S F Ⓕ						I	I	I
I Infertile S Semi Fertile F Fertile Ⓕ Peak Mucus	Verbal Description						Dry	Dry	Dry
Cervix f firm s soft	f s						f	f	f
	●●•∘○○						•	•	•
	I S F						I	I	I
Minor Indicators	O S B F E								
Disturbed/ill	D								
Made Love/Sexual Contact	L								
Fertility Assessment	X/								

Chart 9 – An Anovulatory Cycle

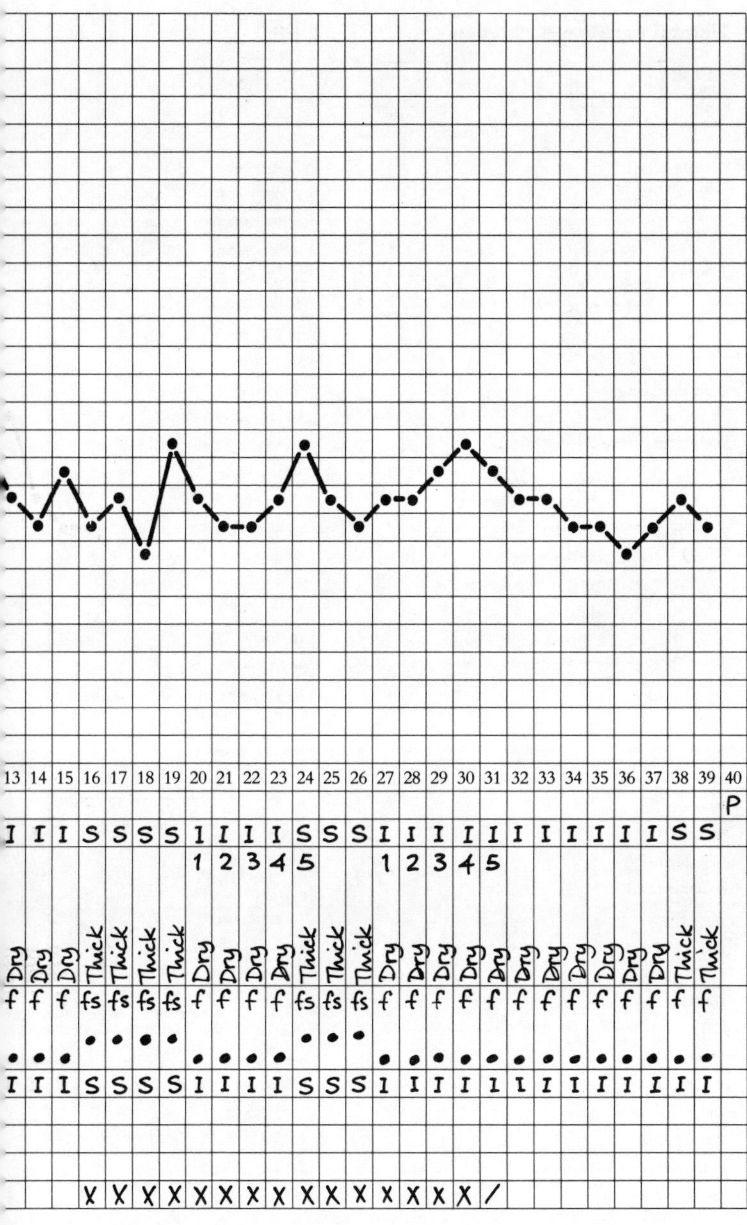
13 14 15 16 17 18 19 20 21 22 23 24 25 26 27 28 29 30 31 32 33 34 35 36 37 38 39 40
P
I I I S S S S I I I I S S S I I I I I I I I I I I S S
1 2 3 4 5 1 2 3 4 5
Dry Dry Dry Thick Thick Thick Thick Dry Dry Dry Dry Thick Thick Thick Dry Dry Dry Dry Dry Dry Dry Dry Dry Dry Dry Thick Thick
f f f fs fs fs fs f f f f fs fs fs f f f f f f f f f f f f f
I I I S S S S I I I I S S S I I I I I I I I I I I I I
X X X X X X X X X X X X X X X /

Natural Fertility Awareness

Chart No: [ ] Year: [ ]

Usual time of taking temperature [ ]

Last 6–12 cycles { Shortest: **24** / Longest: **32**

This cycle length: [ ]

Shortest Cycle – 20 **4**

Minor Indicators
O Ovulation pain
S Blood spotting
B Breasts tender or sore
F Feeling of fullness/heaviness
E Emotional upset

Temperature Rise in Previous Cycle: (YES)/NO

Name: ....

Date								
37.25	99.3							
37.20	99.2							
37.15	99.1							
37.10	99.0							
37.05	98.9							
37.00	98.8							
36.95	98.7							
36.90	98.6							
36.85	98.5							
36.80	98.4							
36.75	98.3							
36.70	98.2							
36.65	98.1							
36.60	98.0							
36.55	97.9							
36.50	97.8							
36.45	97.7							
36.40	97.6	•						
36.35	97.5							
36.30	97.4		•		•			•
36.25	97.3			•				
36.20	97.2					•	•	
36.15	97.1							
36.10	97.0							
36.05	96.9							
36.00	96.8							

	Code	1	2	3	4	5	6	7
	Day	1	2	3	4	5	6	7
Period	P	P	P	P	P	P		
Mucus I Infertile S Semi Fertile F Fertile Ⓕ Peak Mucus	I S F Ⓕ						I	I
	Verbal Description						Dry	Dry
Cervix f firm s soft	f s						f	f
	●●●○○◯						●	●
	I S F						I	I
Minor Indicators	O S B F E							
Disturbed/ill	D							
Made Love/Sexual Contact	L							
Fertility Assessment	X/							

Chart 10 – A Cycle Indicating a Probable Pregnancy

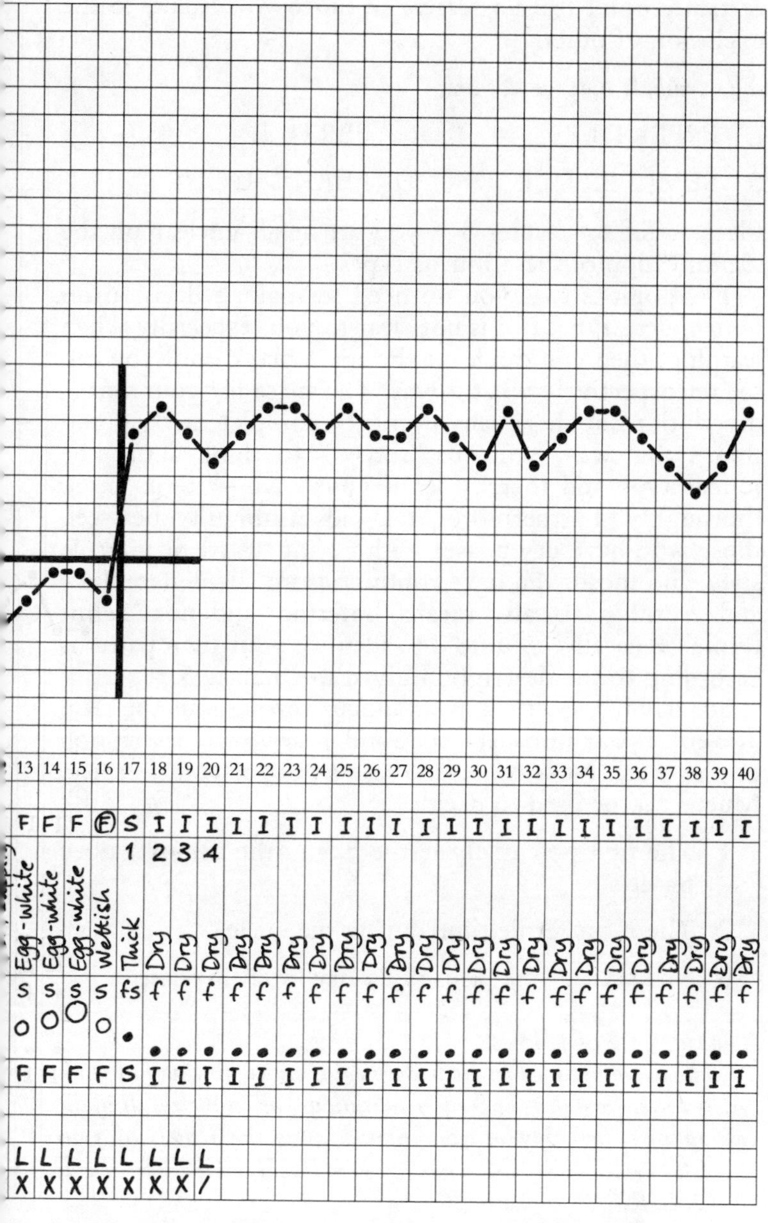
13 14 15 16 17 18 19 20 21 22 23 24 25 26 27 28 29 30 31 32 33 34 35 36 37 38 39 40
F F F F S I I I I I I I I I I I I I I I I I I I I I I I
1 2 3 4
Egg-white
Egg-white
Egg-white
Wettish
Thick
Dry
s s s s fs f f f f f f f f f f f f f f f f f f f f f f f
F F F F S I I I I I I I I I I I I I I I I I I I I I I I
L L L L L L L L
X X X X X X X /

are already familiar with them. Our chart does let you use any letters, symbols or colours that you like and we certainly don't feel possessive of our own system, to the exclusion of others.

The symbols that we use are:

I INFERTILE F FERTILE

S SEMI-FERTILE Ⓕ PEAK MUCUS

Please refer to chapter 5 if you are at all unclear on the identification of these mucus types.

The point is that you do need to make a decision on your mucus type. If it is not clear to you, especially when learning, then you can leave the space blank until you can see retrospectively what it was. The space for your verbal description should, in any event, be completed. By doing things this way, you are "forced" to think about the mucus type and thereby learn your own patterns more thoroughly. Furthermore, it avoids ambiguity between those who have dry phases with no mucus (their infertile state) and those who have continuous mucus, where flaky and crumbly actually means 'Infertile' and not 'Semi-fertile'! Basically, you need to identify your own patterns according to the description given in Chapter 5.

So, having observed your mucus throughout the day, you enter your alphabetic code and your verbal description on the chart. Now comes the assessment of your fertility. Mucus can be used to decide:

1. The first potentially fertile day in the pre-ovulatory phase.
2. The most fertile time during the cycle.
3. The start of the post-ovulatory infertile phase.

The rules are as follows:
1. The pre-ovulatory fertile phase begins on the first day of semi-fertile or fertile mucus or cervix indications, or on the result of the calculation "first day of your period, plus the length of your shortest cycle, less 20 days", WHICHEVER IS THE SOONER.

We use a stringent calendar calculation to give us the same

degree of contraceptive safety as can be achieved in the post-ovulatory infertile phase. The *shortest cycle minus 20* is an outside calculation, especially when combined with mucus observations. Many users prefer a calculation of *shortest cycle minus 18* to determine the start of the fertile phase, unless there is already semi-fertile mucus.

OVIA (see next chapter) actually uses *both* calculations, indicating a gradually less infertile assessment between the 'shortest cycle minus 20' and the 'shortest cycle minus 18'. Because it can accurately indicate the truer state of affairs, i.e. a *less* infertile state, though not actually fertile, *OVIA* starts the pre-ovulatory fertile phase on the shortest cycle minus eighteen or whenever mucus or cervical indications are no longer infertile.

During your period, since mucus cannot be observed, you can use a *shortest day minus 20* calculation to determine your earliest possible fertile day. However, there are two possible ways in which you could become pregnant by making love during your period:

(a) If it isn't really your period at all, but only mid-cycle bleeding, perhaps during an abnormally long cycle. So you need to be sure that it really is your period (did you observe a temperature shift?)

(b) If you had an earlier ovulation (and subsequently shorter cycle) than you have ever had previously, *and* the sperm had an abnormally long life, or it was towards the end of a long period. The point being that until your period has ended, you can't observe the mucus to check that an early ovulation is not on its way.

The next rule is:

2. *You are at your most fertile around the time when your mucus and cervix are in their most fertile condition.*

Your "most fertile mucus" can be determined from your own past experience. There is some discussion of this in Chapter 5, so we won't repeat it here.

Finally, the rule for the first day of the post-ovulatory infertile phase, is:

3. The post-ovulatory infertile phase begins on the third morning of a sustained temperature shift where all three temperatures are greater than any of those taken on the previous six days, or the fourth evening after the last day of fertile mucus (Peak Mucus), or fertile cervix signs, WHICHEVER IS THE LATER.

Peak Mucus is identified retrospectively as the day after which there is a (usually sudden) return to the semi-fertile or infertile condition. It is the last day of fertile mucus. Remember that it may not have been the day of the most copious or the most fertile-looking mucus, but it will normally be demonstrated by a sharp change.

Various possible mucus recordings are given on Charts 2–10, which should be studied with the following notes:

Chart 2 shows the standard mucus pattern of dry or no mucus, moving to white and thick, becoming moist and finally wet; then a sharp reversal to no mucus or dry for the remainder of the cycle except the last three days before the period starts when mucus again appears as the cervix begins to open to allow the menstrual flow. Note that we assess day eight as fertile because of the rule: *Shortest cycle minus 20 equals the first day of the fertile phase,* though in this case the mucus and cervix both indicated infertility. We are just being particularly safe.

Chart 3 shows how this would appear in a woman whose basic pattern of infertile conditions are not totally dry, but are a dryish mucus.

Chart 4 is more or less the same as 2, but with different verbal descriptions. Note that 'flu has not affected the mucus, in this instance, and that making love would mean leaving a blank space for the day after. If using mucus and temperature only, one would miss a day in order to observe the mucus again. If checking the cervix too, this would allow one to still check one's infertile condition and make love in confidence.

Chart 5 has no mucus recorded, so only the post-ovulatory infertile phase can be considered as safe.

Chart 6 shows how the mucus pattern can clarify an unclear temperature rise. All the same, it is safer to wait until the temperature rise is identifiable.

Chart 7 shows a very short cycle.

Chart 8 shows a very long cycle.

Chart 9 shows the patchy mucus of an anovulatory cycle, perhaps characteristic of the individual, perhaps due to stress. From the mucus, we can determine when fertility is rising and if wanting to avoid conception, simply give all such times a wide berth of at least five days, to see what happens next.

Chart 10 shows a probable pregnancy. We have marked with an 'L' in the respective column when making love could have resulted in pregnancy, but note that had this been the case, the mucus recordings on the next day could not have been so easily observed, due to the presence of seminal fluid and vaginal secretions.

Charting Your Cervical Changes

As with the mucus observations, cervix observations are made only after your period has ended. There is less variation amongst the different researchers over how to chart cervical changes than mucus changes, probably because it is really quite clear what to chart. We have again made a three letter key, as follows:

I	Infertile	Low, closed, firm, dimple-like, dry, gritty.
S	Semi-fertile	Changing towards fertile indications, sticky, starting to open, rising a little.
F	Fertile	Soft, ripe, open, high, sticky, slippery.

If in doubt, leave the space blank, it may clarify itself the next day with the benefit of hindsight.

The chart has two rows. Firstly, a wide one in which to indicate the openness or otherwise of the os, its position in the abdomen as discovered by internal observation and whether it is firm or soft ('f' or 's'). Secondly, a narrow one in which to record I, S or F as above.

The rules for interpreting the cervix are the same as

those for the mucus. If there is any conflict, then for the sake of safety, take the most fertile indication as your guide. As we pointed out earlier, the mucus comes from the cervix and travels down by gravity to the vaginal entrance. So the cervix may be indicating a more fertile condition than the mucus at the labia.

This set of charts indicates the way the cervix is likely to behave under the circumstances already allocated to these charts and no further notes are required. Please refer back to the notes for the mucus charts.

Cutting Corners

Once you are *absolutely sure* that you understand your fertility indications, and if, over a period of not less than six consecutive cycles:

1. Your cycles are of regular and more or less predictable length,
2. Your time of ovulation is more or less constant,
3. You are happy to restrict love-making to the post-ovulatory infertile phase to avoid conception,

Then:

1. You need not record the cervical mucus or cervix condition
2. You can skip a number of days at the start and end of the cycle, so that you can begin recording in time to detect the temperature shift and stop soon after it has been detected. *OVIA* will be able to tell you itself how many days you may skip, but if charting, or wanting to make your own decision, then the rule is:

Begin recording at least eight days before the earliest previous temperature shift during your last six to twelve cycles. You can stop recording after at least three days of undisturbed, raised temperature.

We start at least eight days before the earliest previous temperature shift to allow for any disturbed days and an even earlier temperature rise than ever previously recorded. Amongst the thousands of records we examined from Professor John Marshall's research in London, there were numerous series of charts from people who, knowing that their cycles were regular, charted only enough days to be sure of identifying their temperature shift. One could see that sometimes they got caught out by starting their recording too late, or by disturbed temperatures (caused by cold or 'flu) when they had only a few days to record before the shift.

If you want to identify the early pre-ovulatory infertile days, then you must record all the indicators until the post-ovulatory phase has been definitely identified. You can stop recording after at least three days of undisturbed, raised temperature.

However, even if you are not recording your mucus and/or cervical indicators, we recommend that you observe them and, to avoid pregnancy, don't make love if there are any indications of fertility.

Minor Indicators, Making Love and Other Factors

These again can be indicated on the chart in the row provided. Any other comment can be written in on the temperature chart or in the *disturbances* row. Making love can also be marked in the relevant place ('L'). We suggest the following codes for the minor indicators:

O Ovulation pain
S Blood spotting or discharge
B Breasts tender or sore
F Feeling of fullness or heaviness down below
E Emotional upset (more than usual!)

Fertility Assessment Summary

Finally, as you enter each record, you can make your assessment, according to the various rules. Fertility may be entered as an 'X' in the relevant square with a '/' (half an 'X') for the final day of the fertile phase, since this will be identified during the course of the day. You can make love safely, therefore, whenever you don't make a fertile assessment.

The rules may be summarized and repeated as follows:

1. *The time of your period is never totally safe for making love because you cannot observe the mucus or cervix indicators.*
2. *After your period, you are in the pre-ovulatory infertile phase until the pre-ovulatory fertile phase begins.*
3. *The pre-ovulatory fertile phase begins on the first day of semi-fertile or fertile mucus or cervix indications, or on the result of the calculation "first day of your period, plus the length of your shortest cycle, less 20 days", WHICHEVER IS THE SOONER.*
4. *You are at your most fertile around the time when your mucus and cervix are in their most fertile condition.*
5. *The post-ovulatory infertile phase begins on the third morning of a sustained temperature shift, all three of which are greater than any of the temperatures taken on the previous six days, or on the fourth evening after the last day of fertile mucus (Peak Mucus) or fertile cervix signs, WHICHEVER IS THE LATER.*
6. *The post-ovulatory infertile phase lasts until your period starts.*

This then is a complete and simple explanation of how to enter information onto your chart and make an accurate assessment of your level of fertility. If you find it confusing, you may find that the second method described in the next chapter is a clearer and neater way of doing things.

CHAPTER 8

Graded Fertility Assessment – Using Ovia

Human Factors and Reliability

The second and most modern method of assessing fertility is to use a small computer-based instrument, *OVIA*, created by the Wholistic Research Company of Cambridge. The authors, along with Robin Langridge of Cambridge's renowned Computer Aided Design Centre, have devised an objective and automatic assessor of your fertility that only requires you to type in (with one or two fingers only – no typing experience necessary) the information that you would otherwise put onto your chart.

While it would have been possible to write a 'quick' piece of computer programming (the software), fudging over many important aspects of fertility assessment, *OVIA's* software has, in fact, taken a great deal of time to research, write and test. Various aspects of *OVIA* have, or course, been protected under the international copyright and patent laws, the investment in research and development being rather too heavy to hand out on a free for all basis!

The thinking behind the creation of *OVIA* is really twofold:

1. Difficulties With Charting

Most women only have experience of their own cycles and because nature is not always as standard as textbook descriptions, it can sometimes become confusing as to how to interpret a chart. *OVIA's* 'intelligence' is built on the experience of thousands of women and their charts, and it can readily interpret and make assessments that might otherwise be interpreted incorrectly.

2. Inaccurate User Assessements

It is often not generally appreciated that *all* methods of contraception have a failure rate due to the method itself, even when the method is practised or used perfectly. For example – according to surveys – vasectomy, the combined Pill and multi-indicator natural methods, all have an effectiveness of 99% or more. The condom, diaphragm with spermicides, the IUD, the mini-Pill and the mucus indicator on its own have an effectiveness of around 97%. Other methods have less than 90%. However, when the methods are not correctly used or applied, then the failure rate is higher.

One of the problems in this respect with natural fertility indicators (though it should really be considered a plus factor), is that the users are required to take more *responsibility* on themselves than with any other method. They must thoroughly understand how to *observe* the indicators correctly and then they must know how to *interpret* them. And they must also be fully *motivated to act* according to their assessment. It is on these last two accounts that *OVIA* can help considerably.

OVIA's Graded Assessment

OVIA's assessment is objective and based on an experience which it would be well nigh impossible for the average person to attain. The methods and rules described in previous chapters of this book are, of course, based on the research experience of many years. However, *OVIA* incorporates a number of additional rules for contraceptive safety that are rarely taken into account by users of natural fertility awareness methods, simply because too many rules become confusing to the human mind, and therefore counterproductive, while *OVIA's* little computer just gobbles them up!

These additional rules are mostly related to extensive cross-checking between the various fertility indicators, as well as slowly compiling a personal history of your cycles for use in its current assessment. As a consequence of this cross-checking, *OVIA* is able to make a *graded assessment* of your probable fertility, in the following manner:

OVIA has a four line display, with a maximum of 24 characters per line. This display is divided into two parts: one in which you communicate with *OVIA* and the other in which *OVIA* gives you your fertility assessment – see figure 5.

Monday Day 6, Morning Temp. (OC)?—	—OVIA— PRE-OVUL INFERTILE ♥♥♥♥♥♥♥♥
Communication Area	*Fertility Assessment Area*

Figure 5

We will come to the left hand *OVIA Communication Area* later, but just now, examine the right hand, *OVIA Fertility Assessment Area*. It is constituted as follows:

	Contents	**Meaning**
Line 1	—*OVIA*—	Heading
Line 2	PERIOD	You still have your period.
	PRE-OVUL	You are in the pre-ovulatory phase – fertile or infertile.
	OVULING	Ovulation has or is about to occur.
	POST-OVU	You are in the post-ovulatory infertile phase.
	PREGNANT	You could be pregnant.
Line 3	FERTILE	You are in the fertile phase.
	INFERTILE	You are in an infertile phase.
Line 4	♥♥♥♥♥♥♥♥	A row of up to eight ♥'s which tells you *how* fertile or infertile you are.

The fertility assessment rules are much simpler than chart interpretation.

1. *For those wanting to totally avoid pregnancy: only make love when you have a five heart, (♥♥♥♥♥), or more, INFERTILE assessment.*

This will give you the 99% success rate achievable by the Pill and *barrier methods* of contraception. Normally, this means during the first few days of your cycle and in the post-ovulatory infertile stage. If you occasionally or frequently have short cycles of 20 days or less, then only the post-ovulatory phase will be considered as safe.

2. *For those who don't really mind if they get pregnant, but would prefer it if they don't just yet: then any INFERTILE rating is all right.*
   This will still give you a high probability of not getting pregnant.

3. *For those wanting to achieve a pregnancy, the best times are from a three heart, (♥♥♥), or more FERTILE assessment.*
   If you want to conserve your energies, then wait until the assessment is four, five or more hearts.

During the pre-ovulatory part of a cycle, *OVIA's* graded assessment lets you know exactly where you stand. For example, during your period you will never get more than an INFERTILE four heart, (♥♥♥♥), assessment, because the mucus cannot be checked. After the end of your period, up to an INFERTILE five heart, (♥♥♥♥♥), assessment will be indicated if you have infertile mucus or cervix indications before the 'shortest cycle minus 21' defines the outside limit of the calendar calculation's safe period. The pre-ovulatory FERTILE phase starts whenever mucus or cervix indicators are anything other than infertile or whenever the 'shortest cycle minus 18' reaches zero. Prior to that, however, but after the 'shortest cycle minus 21' you will be given an INFERTILE three or four heart, (♥♥♥♥) assessment, assuming that the mucus and/or cervix indications are infertile. You don't need to be able to follow all this exactly, because the results of this cross-checking are displayed simply as FERTILE or INFERTILE with the number of hearts showing the degree, but the essence of it is that *OVIA* is able to portray to you in a graphic and direct manner the changing tides of your fertility.

Human Factors in Natural Birth Control

The value of this *graded assessment* is to aid your decision making about whether or not you really want to avoid or achieve pregnancy, as well as in giving you a more accurate and definitive way of knowing your *degree* of fertility at any one time. All researchers into natural fertility awareness and indeed all methods of contraception, talk of two key human factors that influence the effectiveness of the methods. These we may identify as: *motivation* and *clarity of intention*. If you watch people trying to cross a busy road (where there are no pedestrian crossings!), you will notice that there are at least two motives in the minds of the pedestrians. One is the fear of being injured; the other is the desire to reach the other side. In addition to this, there will also be other factors on a person's mind, surfacing as half-formed, or even stronger thoughts, while he (or she) tries to get across. Now, any of these can be predominant, or can suddenly *become* predominant! Thus, the person may suddenly dash across, causing cars to brake, when he sees his girlfriend or the last bus arriving – or whatever. Or the fear of injury may keep them on the kerb for many minutes, waiting for the ultra-safe moment. Or they may be so distracted by their other thoughts that they walk or run out in front of the traffic and get hurt. Or they just stand on the kerb in a reverie! We can all, I think, identify with these states of mind. We have all experienced similar states to one degree or another, on a regular day to day basis. It is normal human behaviour!

What also happens, quite frequently, is that first one thought and then another becomes predominant, to the extent that the person *dithers*. They are *undecided*. And it is this *oscillating motivation* or *lack of clear intention* that often leads to disaster. You may have experienced driving in a large urban complex of fast moving vehicles and flyovers where you don't know the way. While everyone else moves along within the general fast flow of traffic, you alone are moving slowly and unsurely. Indeed you are a danger on the roads both to yourself and others at that time! But if you go ahead and stay at the same speed as all the rest, you may make a wrong decision and get lost.

Lack of clear intention and in this example, *lack of knowledge and experience,* too, can become your downfall.

Similarly, with natural methods of birth control. It is often quite surprising how many couples do not know for sure whether they want a baby at any given time. They may have differing points of view which have remained unresolved, so that no clear, joint decision has been made. This is especially true if they know that they want a child, but can't make up their minds as to when. There may be other factors too. Perhaps the husband does not fully understand or wish to co-operate with his wife with regard to her fertile or infertile times. He may take offence, through his lack of understanding, and his wife gives in to avoid upsetting him – and takes a chance on getting pregnant. He may think that it is her way of rejecting him. Or the couple may have had a fight and are making up again – now how does the wife say "no" at this point if they are moving towards making love? The whole fight may blow up again. Or maybe, the couple just get carried away in their desire for each other and with no clear decision having been made on getting pregnant, they don't consider the long term consequences and responsibilities of a child.

There are many possibilities. It is important, therefore, that a couple discuss their feelings and desires and come to a joint and positive decision. They may *decide* to remain undecided – especially if they want to have a baby and don't *really* mind when it happens, though taking reasonable precautions to avoid fertile phases. But clarity, there must be if you want to avoid pregnancy. Indecision is a sure recipe for an unplanned baby.

The problem is, of course, that one may on rational or co-operative grounds make a joint decision and yet have a desire, perhaps almost unrecognised or subconscious, which would lead in the opposite direction. You may decide not to have a baby and yet one or other of you would, in their heart, be very happy if one came along.

Many of us are not aware how powerful these subconscious desires and attitudes can be in determining both the things we do, the decisions we make – especially the spontaneous ones – and indeed, the things that happen to us, apparently through no agency of our own.

It is readily understandable, therefore, how a slightly ambiguous fertility chart can be *unconsciously* interpreted to suit one's inner desires and an unplanned pregnancy result. Or you simply can't wait to make love, when you know that there is a risk of pregnancy. It is this kind of *user error* that lowers the actual level of contraceptive success with any of the methods.

Human Factors and OVIA

The point is that *OVIA* makes the fertility assessment *objectively*. It doesn't have human emotions and subconscious desires and motives! Your husband may argue with you, but he (probably) won't argue with a computer! He may even get interested and help you with taking your temperature or entering the information. Most couples, of course, do co-operate fully and this is how it should be. But with *OVIA's* simple rule : INFERTILE 5-hearts (♥♥♥♥♥), or more means you are as safe as the method will allow (about 99% according to surveys) and INFERTILE 4-hearts, (♥♥♥♥), means that you are as safe as the pre-ovulatory methods after the shortest cycle minus 21 day has passed will allow (the surveys say 97%), there is no room for making a mistake due to the emotions or desires of the moment. If you decide to ignore it, then you know the level of risk you are taking.

For these reasons then, we feel that it is quite possible that *OVIA* will remove a fair degree of user error from natural methods of fertility awareness and represents a significant advance on the older methods of charting.

Modern Technology and Natural Living

There will, one imagines, always be some folk who do not like the idea of having a "computer in the bedroom". Well, firstly, let us say that *OVIA* does not look like a computer – it is more like a calculator. And then the manufacturers have done their best to beautify it, in a simple way. Furthermore, it is very simple and easy to use. The fact that it contains a computer is really immaterial. A computer is simply the right tool for the job – just as computers are used in all areas of technology – the telephone system, electricity, TV and radio broadcasting, even motors cars, washing machines, some modern cookers, at school – not to mention in the writing and printing of this book. We all use technology directly or indirectly, most of which we do not understand nor need to understand other than in our ability to use it. One of the authors (John) had a new car for two months before he even discovered how to open the bonnet (or hood, if you are American) – with an instrument panel before him, there was no need to look inside!

What people are probably objecting to when they spurn the use of modern technology is its intrusion into their personal life or its disharmony with nature. *OVIA* does neither of these. It is designed by people who have both a knowledge of high technology and a love of the harmonious and natural. The theme of the twenty-first century will have to become *A Harmony of Science and Nature* if man or at least his present social structure and "civilization", is to survive. Technology must become a helper to nature, not working to pollute or disturb the natural ecological balance for selfish ends. The law of cause and effect is too powerful for man to get away with self-interested disturbance and destruction of his planet's resources for too long.

This negative feed back has already made him clean up some of his messes. The smogs of Victorian and post-Victorian industrialized London which killed so many are now a thing of the past. But we have created many other environmental problems to which solutions must be found. Overpopulation is interesting in that is has both positive and negative aspects. It is the result of much fine and sustained research, over many decades, to understand and eliminate those factors which historically have decimated sections of our population – disease, famine, war and natural disasters being the most common. Now, the solution has to be found and applied: birth control, natural – or otherwise.

Using OVIA

On a day-to-day basis, *OVIA* is very simple to use and understand. Full operating instructions are given in the manufacturer's manual, so there is no need to go into explicit details here. Basically, you type into *OVIA* the same information that you would otherwise indicate on a chart – your temperature, your mucus and your cervical indicators, the latter two being optional. Other details are entered whenever relevant – the start and end of your period, if you were ill or the recording was disturbed, if you were late or early with your recording, how late or early, if you made love (this is optional), if you forgot to make a record, if you are unsure of some fertility indicator and so on. *OVIA* communicates with you via a dialogue, asking for your basal body temperature, your mucus and cervical signs, plus – if relevant – any of the other details listed above. You type in the answer, using one finger, just as you would use a calculator, all this taking place in the *OVIA Fertility Assessment Area,* (see figure 5). And then *OVIA* gives you its updated fertility assessment as we explained earlier, says: THANKS, BYE! and signs off until you next switch on. It's all very simple and automatic, and you can consult *OVIA* at any time during the day (or night) if you forget your last assessment.

When you first switch on *OVIA*, it goes through an initial sequence with you, asking for the lengths of your longest and shortest cycles over the last year (if in doubt, you type 21 and 40) and which fertility indicators you wish to record. To begin with, if you are new to Natural Fertility Awareness, you would not enter mucus or cervical signs for two or three cycles, until you have come to know your own patterns. However, *OVIA* will be able, if you have normal cycles, to detect and inform you of a temperature shift even during your first cycle and be able to tell you when your post-ovulatory infertile phase begins. If you have had regular length cycles for some time, there will be some INFERTILE five heart, (♥♥♥♥♥), ratings in the pre-ovulatory infertile phase too. *OVIA* keeps a record of the relevant data from your cycles (your 'history') and uses it in future fertility assessment. When you start recording mucus and/or cervix indicators, then you will get a series of accurately graded assessments throughout your full cycle. Access to *OVIA* can also be protected by a personal password for privacy permitting in addition a number of women to use the same device in say a small community or village, making it particularly applicable to the Third World.

Skipping Days and Cutting Corners

The same rules apply as for charting, except that *OVIA* can also tell you how many days you may skip, if you are unsure.

Using OVIA To Become Pregnant

OVIA will tell you, right from the start, when you are at the most fertile point in your cycle. From the presence or absence of a temperature shift, you will know whether or not you are ovulating and once you start recording mucus or cervix indicators, you will know very surely of your most fertile days. There seems to be every reason why *OVIA* will help considerably with infertility problems. Charting has helped, so *OVIA* should be even more helpful. *OVIA* also accepts input from the LH hormone test which predicts ovulation (OVUSTICK) and, correlating it with the other information tells you of the best times to make love in a bid for pregnancy! *OVIA* will also help you economise on the use of the hormone test by telling you when high fertility and, hence, ovulation are approaching.

So all in all, *OVIA* has a lot of things going for it. Obviously, it is not as inexpensive as using a chart. But it has advantages and will last many, many years, which then makes it seem quite cheap in comparison to the on-going costs of most artificial methods of birth control. And finally, if you are so minded, you can also use *OVIA* as a regular calculator and as a small computer, programmable in BASIC.

Wholistic Research Company, whose name and address are at the back of this book, can supply you with all the details of *OVIA*. We think it is definitely worth investigation.

CHAPTER 9

Artificial or Natural Methods of Avoiding a Baby

Reading through the literature and reports available on the different artificial methods of contraception, one is struck by the length of the list of problems and side effects associated with *all* artificial methods of birth control. For technological interruption of the reproductive system, there would seem to be only one positive factor – contraception.

When one reads the literature and talks to people about natural methods however, the nature of the communication is vastly different. Natural methods are seen as part of a way of life, of growing ever closer and in loving communication with one's partner and with nature, of taking time for each other, of co-operation and sharing. The people involved are essentially more wholesome in their outlook on life: they seem less selfish, they care more for the genuine welfare of others. Natural Fertility Awareness is often taught for no charge, if it is not the means of livelihood of the teacher – it is an expression of their concern for the well-being of their fellow humans. They are not super-salesman in what represents, to contraceptive manufacturers, a lucrative market to be milked at almost any cost to the health of the individual, with statistics or lack of research used to cover up the inadequacies from both medical and human emotion points of view.

One cannot help but get a feeling that women are having their natural womanhood and femininity massacred by a wide variety of devices, creams, chemicals and even sterilization. Science cannot create a life, it can only analyse some of its more obvious outward processes. The essence of our being, the complexities of emotion and thought – those qualities which make us know we are alive – are beyond the range of scientific analysis. The side effects, therefore, especially the long term effects, of upsetting any aspect of nature, let alone one of such significance as our procreative systems, can never be fully understood. We do not deny the great advances of technology, but we do make a plea for a harmony of science with nature.

Using natural methods, the positive factors may be summarized:

1. Being in harmony with yourself and with nature means no negative side-effects.
2. You receive a valuable knowledge of your body cycles, useful in other aspects of being alive.
3. You develop a more personal and knowledgeable sense of responsibility concerning sex and pregnancy.
4. Couples are brought together in a more sharing, co-operative and mutual understanding.
5. They can be used for both achieving or avoiding pregnancy, making it true fertility awareness, not just contraception, and therefore of use to a high percentage of couples who have infertility difficulties.

There are a number of good syntheses of surveys of the health hazards and reliability of artificial methods of contraception. The best we have come across is in Dr. Evelyn Billings and Ann Westmore's book *The Billings Method*. We will just list here the reliability ratings and some of the problems associated with these methods. We are purposely not listing the comparative advantages between the methods. We leave that to the responsible decision of the individual. We do not wish to obscure the risk elements involved.

Method	*Reliability*	*Side-effects, problems and comments*
Intra-Uterine Devices. (IUD's)	94–97%	Foreign objects that bounce around, causing irritation, in the womb. Prevents implantation of the fertilized ovum and is really an abortive agent. If pregnancy does result, 30–50% end in a miscarriage. 5–10% of pregnancies are ectopic – within the Fallopian tube resulting in a rupture of the tube and removal by surgery with decreased chances of conception afterwards. Can cause heavy menstruation and possible anaemia. Can perforate the uterine wall requiring a hysterectomy. Can be painful to insert if you have never had a baby and may tear the cervix, which has to be dilated with a mechanical device. Can cause cramping and backache. They lose their effectiveness after a number of years and need to be replaced, normally because nature, not surprisingly, did the best it could and gave the IUD a coating of calcium to make it less irritating. Sometimes they get lost inside and there is a problem getting them out. About 30% of women give up their use with in a year.
Condom	81–97%	A rubber sheath fitting over the man's penis. Aesthetically unappealing and interrupts the spontaneity of love making. Sperm can escape around the top or it can come off altogether.

Method	*Reliability*	*Side-effects, problems and comments*
Diaphragm, with spermicide	64–97%	A dome or cap that covers the cervix. Must be well-fitted by a doctor to be efficient. Reliability depends upon the use of a good spermicide. Spermicides can cause irritation of the vagina and be absorbed into the body. Related to urinary tract infections (cystitis). Disrupts spontaneity. Obscures observation of the mucus.
Honeycap	Unknown	A special kind of more natural diaphragm that is impregnated with honey and can be left in place for days on end without any odour developing, honey being a natural anti-microbe agent. No spermicides are required. We are currently trying to find out more about the reliability of this device, since it seems the best diaphragm we have come across.
Spermicides alone	65–93%	A cream or foam that kills sperm. See above. Sometimes held in a sponge, located within the vagina.
Withdrawal before ejaculation	30–50%	Semen escapes before ejaculation, so the method doesn't work very well. Causes anxiety to the couple and emotional difficulties.
Vasectomy	99% and more	This process involves incisions within the scrotum, (the sac of skin holding the testes), cutting the tubes (vas deferens) which lead from the testes, conveying the sperm to the outside. The

Method	*Reliability*	*Side-effects, problems and comments*
		psychological aspects of this procedure are more or less unavoidable. Men generally feel that they have lost part of their manhood and suffer a loss of self-esteem. About 6% – 10% of those in the U.S.A. want a reversal (which is only very marginally possible) because of divorce and remarriage.
Sterilization	99% and more	This usually involves cutting, electrically burning or tieing the fallopian tubes. An operation is required under local or general anaesthetic. Sometimes the uterus is removed (hysterectomy). The former method can be reversed, but only by the most skillful of surgeons, where the success rate is up to 50%. The physical complications of this procedure can include severe bleeding, infection and ectopic pregnancies in the fallopian tube. Menstrual problems, such as heavy bleeding, vary from between 8% to 25% of sterilized women and the blood supply to the uterus is disturbed in about a third of women, occasionally necessitating a hysterectomy. Severe feelings of guilt, remorse, depression and other emotional disturbances often follow sterilization, as might be expected.
Rhythm Method	86–94%	Simply unreliable because of the uniqueness of each cycle.

Method	*Reliability*	*Side-effects, problems and comments*
Combined Pill	99% or more	Contains synthetic oestrogen and progesterone.
Low Level Combined Pill	94–97%	Contains a lesser amount of the same substances.
Mini-Pill	94–97%	Only contains progesterone.
Morning After Pill	Unknown	For emergency use only. Makes most women feel sick.

The Pill

There are, in fact, over forty different contraceptive pills on the market that inhibit ovulation by suppressing the release of pituitary LH and FSH hormones. They also disrupt the uterine lining (the endometrium) making it incapable of nurturing a fertilized ovum. The unknown or suspected side-effects include: a change in carbohydrate, thyroid, liver and fat metabolism which can also lead to weight gain, fluid retention, headaches, breast tenderness, increased skin pigmentation, increased mucus from cervical glands, cervical erosion, possible lowering of seizure threshold in epileptics, depression, frigidity, decreased confidence, emotional upsets, high blood pressure and heart problems, abnormalities in blood clotting tests, stroke and other forms of thrombosis (blood clots), liver tumours, cancer of reproductive areas including breasts, nausea, reduced levels of Vitamin C and other mineral and vitamin imbalances, and an increased risk of infection especially of the vagina, acne and an oily skin, smaller breasts, breakthrough bleeding.

Women with the following problems are advised not to take the Pill: any family or personal history of breast cancer or of other areas of the reproductive system, thrombosis, angina pectoris (heart pains), diabetes, high blood pressure or cholesterol, migraines, kidney or gall bladder diseases, epilepsy. Cigarette smokers have a five times greater likelihood of heart disease if taking the Pill as well, and ten times the probability of those neither smoking nor taking the Pill (this information comes from the American Food and Drug Administration). The FDA also insist that all contraceptive pills supplied in the U.S.A. come with two foolscap pages of side-effect warnings. Those with irregular cycles are advised against taking it and all users are advised to avoid pregnancy until their cycles become regular after they come off the Pill. In some cases, this may take many months and a very small percentage never return to fertility. After pregnancy, there is an increase in foetal abnormalities, in miscarriages if the women go right onto the Pill and the quantity and quality of breast milk is also effected and the hormones are found in the milk.

There is concern that the Pill, which has only been in use for less than twenty years, may also cause genetic abnormalities in the offspring of those who have taken it. These children are only just reaching child-bearing age and although they may not themselves show any defects, at least so far, their problems may be compounded when two of these children have their own babies – or it may take further generations for problems to become apparent, by which time the original cause will be lost. Oestrogen and progesterone are powerful chemicals that seem to effect practically all the systems of the body – physical, emotional and mental. Man's image of time is very short and self-interested, while a hundred years is nothing in the history of the earth. One wonders, in this respect, whether the general increase in cancer and heart disease has any foundation in the continual use of artificial medicines and drugs as well as environmental pollution. It seems highly likely.

Between 33% and 50% of women give up using the Pill within one year and a 1978 study by the British Family Planning Association showed that half a million women had stopped taking the Pill in that year alone – about 14% of all the users.

Forgetting to take the Pill for just a day can result in an LH surge leading to an immediate ovulation, and a resultant pregnancy with possible complications. With the Mini-Pill, if you forget for longer than three hours, then pregnancy might follow. With the regular Pill you have about twelve hours. With the low level Pill, studies have indicated that ovulation would seem to be prevented perhaps only 50% of the time, meaning that the Pill is acting as an early abortive agent. With the Mini-Pill (progesterone only), ovulation may be occurring 60% of the time.

The full effects of any hormone or chemical within the body can never be fully worked out or described. Most of the major outward and easily observable hormone functions may have been recorded, though even that cannot be said categorically. What is considered as unimportant today may be seen as essential in the light of fresh evidence. Take the instance of the pineal gland, a small endocrine gland situated within the brain cavity at the rear base of the third ventricle. This organ, which becomes calcified soon after puberty, was long thought by conventional medicine to have no function in later life. Recent research, however, has shown that the pineal gland produces a number of biologically active compounds and is also probably stimulated by light received from the eye, via an indirect neural connection in the spinal cord. Its functions at a biochemical/neurological level are still far from understood, but what is known is that it is connected with the 24-hour circadian rhythm that wakes us up and makes us tired and a good many other things besides. It also has a role to play in seasonal depressions or "mid-winter blues".

Our point is that to play around with the patterns of life is bound to create effects in other areas that may be either too subtle to be immediately noticed, recorded, or be personally aware of, or that will take several or even many years, perhaps generations, to become apparent. By which time it will probably be too late to reverse the damage.

Reliability of Natural Methods

We have, throughout our book, given indications of reliability on the various indicators, according to studies and surveys undertaken. To summarize these, we can say once again that the use of the temperature shift to determine the post-ovulatory infertile phase has an accredited success rate of 99% in avoiding pregnancy.

Regarding the use of the mucus indicators by themselves, a 1976 Australian survey, amongst women who had been well taught, gave the cervical mucus indicators a contraceptive success rating of 97%, *when used on their own*.

However, the World Health Organization have come up with figures of 87%, where the method has either not been thoroughly understood or taught, or where motivation is lacking. In the Fairfield trial of 1977, a rating of 99% was given to users of the temperature indicators linked to an accurate calendar calculation to predict the early infertile phase.

No fullscale surveys have yet been done on combined methods, using all the available indicators, but it would seem clear that the success rate will be 99% or greater, where the methods are practised with knowledge, diligence and understanding. This, of course, compares favourably with the Combined Pill and sterilization or vasectomy, but without any risk of side effects.

In this respect, we feel that the *OVIA* graded fertility assessment system will perhaps prove more reliable, and certainly easier, than charting, because it is quite objective and unequivocal, and can take into account all the factors. It is not likely to be swayed by sexual desire or other subconscious or conscious motives in its interpretations and its "five hearts or more" rule gives you the opportunity to choose for maximum contraceptive safety at all times.

Conclusions

Of all these artificial methods, if you need to use them, a barrier method would seem to be the least harmful. But we must again point out the sense of personal well-being that comes from working with nature. Artificial methods of contraception break the flow of the Life Force, they disturb the subtle energy pathways within our body and our being. To understand our bodies and to take responsibility for our own welfare is something few people accept. We need to become "individuated" as Jung put it – loving, wholesome, vibrant, positive human beings using our intelligence and working in harmony with the natural laws.

CHAPTER 10

The Past and the Future

Natural understanding of the fertility cycle is not something new. Some of the methods now used may be new, in keeping with our more technological culture, but technology and literacy are not equatable with human inner development and mutual, loving understanding. There have been many tribes, communities and cultures in touch with the natural rhythms of nature where the natural flow is closely mirrored in their lifestyle. In fact, probably all the "earth peoples" – from Australian aboriginees to African bushmen – now practically obliterated from our world, come into this category, as well as more sophisticated cultures. Biologists call this natural rhythm-linkage: *bio-entrainment,* and acknowledge its existence in all living creatures, the most obvious being the twenty-four hour circadian rhythm of day and night, to which we are all entrained.

The word "menstruation" itself comes from the Latin word "menses", meaning one month or a period of a month, and refers to the more or less average cycle of a month between a woman's periods. This association with the moon is not so off-beat as it may seem. Many species are entrained to lunar cycles. The marine biologist, Dr. Bob Johannes, studied the natural history of the Palau Islands, discovering that more than fifty local species of fish have their spawning cycles entrained to the moon. Lunar entrainment has also been observed in land-based creatures and fresh water fish, so it is not necessarily a tidal or gravitational phenomenon.

Perhaps when living closer to nature, human communities are more readily locked on to the lunar as well as other natural cycles? In this respect Edmond Dewan, an American biophysicist has some interesting evidence. Reasoning that primates would be safest ovulating at full moon, when they were less vulnerable to surprise attack by predators, he and a colleague, Dr John Rock, at the Rock Reproductive Clinic in Roxbury, Massachussetts, requested nineteen women with menstrual irregularity to sleep with the light on from days 14 to 17 of their cycles. They reported that most of the women were able to regularize their cycles *immediately* and several of them later became pregnant after having had infertility problems before that.

If you want to try this out, you should first of all make sure that your room is dark at night, not lit up by street lamps or passage lights. Then, during days fourteen to seventeen of your cycle, keep an ordinary table lamp on the floor at the base of your bed. Dewan used a 100W bulb, though a less intense bulb may also suffice. And if you do try this, do please let us know the result, whether it is positive or negative.

Dewan's explanation is that light can affect the pituitary along a direct link from the retina of the eye, through the central nervous system. And the pituitary, we know, has a direct link with the ovaries through the hormonal sequence. Perhaps, reasons Dewan, light as well as the rise in ovarian oestrogen, also helps to stimulate the release of LH from the pituitary?

In fact, Louise Lacey, in her book: *Lunaception*, provides a full explanation of how to use lunar cycles to predict ovulation. Fertility rites in ancient cultures have frequently been related to lunar cycles, so there is plenty of grounds for further research. It would not be the first time that the wheel has been re-invented.

With regard to the effect of light on the reproductive system, there is certainly evidence linking the pineal gland to the body rhythms as well as to the stimulus of light. Tests with rats have shown that the onset of puberty is earlier when exposed to prolonged periods of light, which could possibly be one of the explanations behind the earlier onset of *menarche* in young girls, nowadays. Menarche is another word with lunar connections – *Men* being the Greek for moon, and *arche,* beginning. Traditionally, this is almost totally ascribed to better nutrition, which no doubt has plenty to do with it. However, all modern children are more exposed to light than in previous centuries and ages.

A Czechoslovakian psychiatrist and gynaecologist, Dr. Eugen Jonas, has taken this cyclic aspect of fertility into the realms of astrology. Using the angle, at the moment of birth, between the sun and moon on a geocentric horoscope, Jonas is able to calculate what he calls the *cosmic fertility period*. The correct sun and moon angle come round every 29.53 days, the synodic lunar period and since most women do not have cycles that exactly correspond to this rhythm, the fertile period will move around within the cycle, which of course explains why the rhythm method is so unpredictable. Jonas claims that verifying tests have been made with over 10,000 women volunteers for both the achievement and avoidance of pregnancy. In one year-long test involving 1,252 women, Jonas claims that 97% confirmed the method to be reliable in avoiding pregnancy.

We mention this work here because man has a history of rejecting what he cannot understand today as heresy, but welcoming it with open arms in future times with the benefit of greater knowledge. These methods definitely deserve the respect of further research.

In other cultures, there is evidence of natural birth control being practised. A Central Indian tribe, the Muria, numbering about 200,000, put their boys and girls together in children's dormitories from an early age, where they live and sleep together until marriage. The tribe is harmonious and so are the children. Furthermore, the rate of pre-marital pregnancy is an astonishingly low, 4%. All the girls appear to do is to pray to the local gods at a ceremony before entering the dormitory, to keep them from becoming pregnant. But there is no expectation that a girl will always be prepared to make love and the speculation is that these girls come to know intuitively of their fertile times. It may also have something to do with their mothers and 'aunts' having knowledge of the mucus indications related to ovulation, or that they are naturally linked with the lunar rhythm, or that they are taught to have a natural intuition as to their fertile times. We have come across similar reports amongst African tribes which include a knowledge of the mucus indicators.

More technological approaches to determining the time

of ovulation include devices based on the work of Professor Harold Saxton Burr, described in his book *Blueprint For Immortality*. Burr discovered an electric field around the body that changed according to many internal conditions, both physical, emotional and mental. He also discovered that a peak voltage was distinguishable between two fingers of the hands around the time of ovulation. There have been devices that detect this for the purposes of predicting ovulation, but as far as we know, no statistical evidence has been collected for determining its use in avoiding or achieving conception or on the possible disturbances due to physical conditions and emotional or mental upsets in the user.

As we discussed earlier, the conditions in the vagina – the acidity, salt, sugar and water content – alll change as the cycle progresses. A number of companies therefore are working on products that directly monitor these conditions, using various dipsticks and similar methods.

As we discovered with the Pill, oestrogen and progesterone also affect the vitamin and mineral balance within the body. Research is therefore being conducted into easy identification of substances found in the saliva during the fertility cycle.

There is a further device under development that measures the viscosity of the cervical mucus, another that removes the cervical mucus to measure its volume, and a couple of others that check for a change in the basal body temperature.

There is an inherent problem with removing mucus for testing, in that the mucus has friendly or hostile characteristics towards sperm, and removing it will only tell you what the situation would have been had it been left in place. Moreover, those who are drawn to practise natural fertility awareness, will probably have a deeper approach to life than seeking superficial, symptomatic solutions to everything. Some of these devices seem to take away the personal responsibility and knowledge that is valued by users of natural fertility awareness methods. With only a green light for 'go' and a red light for 'stop' – or its equivalent – the process of gaining knowledge of one's own body is undermined. Both charting and *OVIA*, as the only two genuine means of natural fertility assessment, augment this knowledge.

The other problems underlying all of these are, firstly, that there is always a probability factor associated with fertility. What is required is a graded assessment of what the chances are that you will or will not become pregnant if you make love, both for achieving and avoiding conception. Most of the devices attempt to simplify the process by being definitive, yes or no, while nature seems to have a disinclination to be tied down so rigidly.

Secondly, no two women (or men!) are the same and their own cycles necessarily vary as well. Therefore, some degree of personal acceptance of responsibility and knowledge of one's own body are essential. Natural Fertility Awareness will automatically arise as a possibility in the minds of people who are developing within themselves. The pill-taking pharmaceutically-entrained, millions who are happy with a superficial, symptom-relieving system of dealing with their problems will always want a pill or an easy way out, even if there are long-term side effects. Indeed, since even the concept of inner peace and physical or emotional well-being is often alien to such folk, a few more side-effects to their lifestyle are often hardly noticeable!

CHAPTER 11

Fertility Awareness Under Special Circumstances

Menarche, Coming off the Pill, Childbirth and Breast Feeding, Climacteric, Infertility

These subjects are really each worth a book of their own and we do recommend that you choose some good reading on these topics. The best synopsis that we have found is in *The Billings Method* by Dr. Evelyn Billings and Ann Westmore, though there are many other specialist books. Please consult the information section at the rear of the book.

Our only criticism of *The Billings Method* (using the mucus indicators only) is that the authors quite unnecessarily seem to go out of their way to knock the other natural indicators of fertility – especially the rise in temperature indicator – as if they were the "competition". We are only interested here in the welfare of our fellow human beings and there is no doubt that a *combination* of indicators gives a higher level of contraceptive safety, than the use of one method by itself. This is not to deny the value of the Billings Method; it is just that the statistical evidence puts both the temperature only method and the combined methods ahead of the mucus only (Billings) method, and the temperature rise is often more readily identifiable than Peak Mucus. But it is always up to the individual to make their own informed decision and to take responsibility for the monitoring of their own fertility, with all the unbiased facts in front of them.

Our aim here is just to give some general guidelines on how to assess your fertility during times when the hormonal balance is changing, not to offer advice or information on how best to deal with these times in your life.

Menarche

Menarche is the time in a young girl's life when she has her first period, normally around thirteen, though it can be several years earlier or later. The early cycles for the first year or so are normally anovulatory and often of irregular length. Periods may even be uncomfortable or painful, and relief may be had by consulting a good naturopathic doctor, as well as, if you wish, a gynaecologist. We definitely advise against taking any hormone-based pills for the relief of symptoms, unless as a last resort, since the side-effects on such a young and delicately balanced system would be hard to determine, especially in the long term.

Now is a good time to start learning about fertile and infertile indicators. Perhaps, to begin with, one may observe the mucus. Discover the infertile pattern of mucus – be it none at all (dry) or of thick and whitish nature or whatever is continuous. Then observe how the body is slowly working up towards ovulation – patches of wetter, more fertile mucus are observable from time to time.

Later on, you can make observations of the cervix and temperature. In some so-called 'primitive' cultures, the women were aware of the natural cycles. These things were taught to the young girls by their mothers and 'aunts' of the community. It is really good if the mother is practising Natural Fertility Awareness and teaches her daughters the same principles.

When ovulation does start, it can be early or late within a cycle and here the temperature indicators provide a sure way of knowing if ovulation has taken place.

It is not our place to moralize here, but whatever else a teenager may do, taking the Pill is not a good idea. As we commented earlier, Dr. Anna Flynn told me that she has had young women in her Birmingham Natural Family Planning Centre who went on the Pill at the age of fourteen and coming off it in their early twenties in order to have a baby. They have therefore experienced hardly any regular periods in their lives or the concomitant feminine aspects of a normal menstrual cycle.

One can understand how a doctor may feel caught between a potential teenage pregnancy and the Pill, but this must surely be considered only as an absolutely outside, last ditch solution. It is a symptom of our times that people want to abrogate personal responsibility by taking a pill, or finding a symptom-removing solution for every problem. But the problem, whatever its nature, will always re-surface somewhere else, perhaps in some worse form. You cannot suppress or eliminate energy, it *will* find expression in one way or another and it needs therefore to be consciously and responsibly guided and channelled.

Coming Off The Pill

There are expectancies and uncertainties as might be anticipated in both taking the Pill and in giving it up. Normally, a woman will experience withdrawal bleeding a few days after ceasing to take the Pill, as the endometrium breaks down and is shed. In an American survey conducted by Evrard and his colleagues in 1976, about 30% of women had a regular period about one month later; 60% took up to two months; 8% took up to six months and a further 2% took longer than 6 months.

If you are wanting to conceive, then you should wait for three or four months. Miscarriages are not infrequent in the early months after giving up the Pill, though if you do conceive early and there is no miscarriage, there is said to be no abnormal risk involved in the pregnancy. But you need to give the body time to get back to normal after the somewhat severe disarrangement of its natural functioning.

If you are now wanting to learn about the natural indicators of fertility, you will need to abstain from making love or from genital contact for at least a month or two, or to make love very infrequently during the post-ovulatory infertile phase, because vaginal secretions and seminal fluid will interfere with your mucus observations. We're sorry about that, but in order to become very clear in your mind about the mucus signs, abstinence is best! Remember the long-term benefits and that not making love doesn't mean not being affectionate to each other. This may seem like a tight regime if you have been used to unrestricted love making while on the Pill. However, it is unlikely that you will learn fast enough to be able to use the mucus or cervix signs to pick up imminent ovulation and the temperature indicator may take a couple of months or more to show a rise, since the first cycles are likely to be anovulatory. The more fertile mucus and cervix signs are likely to come and go several times as the body tries to ovulate, before you can observe a Peak Mucus.

In practise, the best way to approach your learning at this stage is to start taking your temperature right away and either charting or entering it into *OVIA*, which has a special mode for coping with such special and long periods of disturbance.

Also, start observing your mucus and cervix. It may take a few months for the mucus to steady into a regular pattern, but what you are looking for here, after your initial withdrawal bleeding is the *continuous pattern*. This may be dry or a continuous thickish, white mucus – heavy or light. This will be your *typical infertile condition* at this stage, though it may change as the excess hormones in your system are slowly released. Make a note of both mucus and – if you are going to learn about it – your cervix condition too. A chart is most helpful while learning mucus and cervix indicators, because you can enter verbal descriptions and compare notes with previous days.

What you are looking for is a *change* towards semi-fertile or fertile mucus or cervix condition, indicating an attempt by the body to ovulate. It will normally last a few days and return to the typical infertile condition as the hormone levels rise and fall.

Since you will be taking your temperature too, when you observe the temperature shift you will know when ovulation has occurred for the first time and will be able to retrospectively determine your Peak Mucus and fertile cervix conditions. Then you can expect your period within 10 to 16 days. You are now on the road to regaining your full fertility. Many women find this a time for great exultance as nature re-establishes her natural balance after being put in a strait-jacket for all that time.

Mid-cycle spotting or bleeding is quite common during your first cycles after giving up the Pill, so be sure that you don't confuse it with your period. If in doubt, wait!

Keep recording your temperature and observing your

four mornings of a temperature shift – adding an extra day if charting or when you get an INFERTILE 5-heart, (♥♥♥♥♥), assessment from *OVIA*. Before ovulation, if you are *absolutely sure* that you have identified your infertile mucus, then you can make love on alternate infertile days. Don't make love on any days when there is a mucus or cervix *change* and wait for four days after you have observed a *change back* to infertile conditions from semi-fertile or fertile. But mistakes can happen here due to bottled up desire, so we ought to repeat that it is best to wait until after your first temperature rise. Just be nice and loving to each other in other ways and wait for the correct time.

Finally, you will probably find that it takes longer for you to positively identify changes in the cervix than in the mucus. This is quite normal. The rule is:

To be safe, you must be sure of your observation.
Don't guess, or hope for the best!

Childbirth and Breastfeeding

Nature gives you a natural period of infertility after childbirth that can extend to many months or even years if breastfeeding. However, ovulation can occur before your first period, so care needs to be taken to avoid pregnancy.

There is a strong link, reflected in the hormone sequences, between infertility and breastfeeding. There are a number of good books on breastfeeding with chapters on associated infertility, but basically, infertility will normally continue for as long as your baby has free and continuous access to your breasts both for feeding and comfort. If you introduce solids before six months or if the breast milk is disturbed, fertility can start to return and you may observe patches of fertile mucus. If you want to continue breast feeding, however, try not to be dismayed or worried, because this in itself can cause the milk to dry up. Instead, keep your baby even closer and let him or her feed whenever desired and you may well find that the return to fertility subsides.

In certain parts of Africa and India, children are regularly suckled up to five years of age which spaces babies quite naturally at four or five year intervals. Babies often become sensitive and upset by an impending return to fertility and may notice it before you do. Perhaps it is hormones in the milk or a change in its constitution or even a more subtle energy connection between you, probably all of these, but it can be reversed by even closer contact with you. Letting baby sleep with you will also help the breast milk to keep coming.

Night feeding, complementary baby foods, a change in feeding patterns, weaning, teething, sickness and so on, all influence the relationship you have with your baby and will affect the milk supply and your return to fertility.

The rule really is:

The closer the contact and motherly nurturing, the longer the milk will last and the more prolonged the period of natural infertility.

When your baby is first born, the last thing you want to be involved with is taking your temperature and so on. If you are already familiar with the fertility indicators, then identify your pattern of continuous infertile mucus, (see Chapter 5) keeping a watchful eye for any change towards fertility. This infertile mucus may be different from your previous pre-pregnancy infertile condition. The cervix too, will almost certainly be different and you will need to reaquaint yourself with its signs. In addition, your fertile mucus may now not be so different from your previous pre-pregnancy semi-fertile mucus. So in essence, you need to re-identify your mucus and cervix patterns. As soon as you see mucus or cervix signs of fertility returning, then you should start taking and recording your temperature once again. Your temperature at this time may quite commonly be erratic and a true temperature shift not so obviously detectable. So if in doubt – don't. If you want to make love before you first identify a temperature shift, then:

Wait until you have had at least two weeks of positively identifiable infertile dryness or infertile unchanging mucus (your new basic infertile pattern).

After that, much the same rules apply as for any time of

changing fertility patterns. These are:

1. *You can make love safely on alternate nights during infertile times, as identified positively by mucus and perhaps, cervical signs.*
2. *Don't make love when you observe any change towards a fertile mucus or cervix.*
3. *Wait four days after a return to the infertile condition.*
4. *If you identify Peak Mucus, then follow the usual rules of waiting until the fourth evening after Peak.*
5. *Avoid making love during any bleeding.*
6. *Start recording your temperature if you haven't already done so, as soon as there are any indications of fertility.*

Since it is a time of change, it is not a bad idea to add an extra day to all the various rules of thumb, or to let *OVIA* indicate the same condition twice, before taking it as safe.

Climacteric and Menopause

The *climacteric* is the time, normally during the late forties, when a woman's fertility is on the decline. The *menopause* is the last menstruation in her life. Under normal circumstances, when menstruation has not happened for one year, then one would not expect any more periods and you will now be unable to conceive. These can be emotional times, when discussion and reading can give much support. Many women find the post-menopausal phase of their life a time for the fulfillment of goals previously put to one side due to the responsibilities of family life.

After the age of forty five, there is a much lesser chance, statistically, of your becoming pregnant. Your cycles become increasingly variable in length. The frequency of anovulatory cycles increases and mucus changes between often long periods of infertile type, interspaced with brief periods of fertile mucus. Recording your temperature will let you know whenever ovulation is occurring, and you may find that your periods continue for months or years after you are infertile.

The guidelines are the same as for the other times of change in one's life, also dealt with previously in this chapter. You need to look for the infertile pattern of mucus and cervix, making love only on alternate days and giving fertile patches a wide berth of three or four days, once they have receded. If ovulation occurs, and you will know that from your temperature shift, then you will move into a genuinely post-ovulatory infertile phase until your next period, twelve to sixteen days later.

Hot flushes are also associated with low levels of oestrogen and are usually associated with a low level of fertility.

Infertility

We have indicated throughout the book where natural fertility awareness can help you achieve pregnancy, so this is not repeated here. It is estimated that 10% to 15% of couples are childless, while wanting to have a baby and about one in six have problems conceiving. With these kinds of figures, we find it truly surprising that doctors are not taught about the natural indicators of fertility in medical school. It would save many heartaches. It seems to be a prevalent myth that the temperature rise heralds imminent ovulation and at least two couples that we know personally (they only told us later), used this method on their doctor's advice, in order to try and get pregnant. In both cases, it took them about ten years.

There are, of course, many reasons – both in the male and the female – for infertility and it is not our intention to describe them here, there being specialist books on the subject by experienced doctors. Natural methods of fertility awareness will, however, tell you when ovulation is imminent (mucus, cervix and the LH OVUSTICK test) and when or if it has occurred (temperature rise). It is always worth seeing a well recommended practitioner of holistic medicine – an acupuncturist, homeopath, herbalist or whatever you prefer – as well as consulting your doctor or gynaecologist. There are more things in heaven and in earth than can be contained in just one approach to bodily problems.

The reasons for infertility can vary from stress, anxiety

and emotional aspects to physiological or anatomical problems with more or less any of the organs involved in the reproductive process, both male and female. In many cases, the problem is not total – only partial – and identification of the (perhaps infrequent) fertile times is of inestimable value.

Dr. Evelyn Billings quotes a report from one such case. A women thought that she was producing no mucus at all, her sensations were always dry. Then, one day, after keeping watch for six months, she saw fertile mucus. She had no doubt about it. They made love and the next day the fertile mucus was gone. Six weeks later, their doctors confirmed that a baby was on its way.

The Last Word

Life is precious to all. And a *good* life. Our relationships and the way we feel on a day to day basis are of tremendous importance to us. We need to feel a sense of well-being and wholesomeness, if we are to be good human beings. A sense of personal responsibility is required. We need to eliminate any tendency to blame others for the ills of the world and in ourselves and others. We need to stand straight, look out at the world with loving confidence from behind our own eyes, to live according to our highest ideals. Humanity desperately needs this. We do not need to join charitable or peace-making organizations or to become ecologists to improve matters in this world. It is good that there are groups and individuals who perform this function and we can help or join if our inclinations are strong enough. But every individual spreads unconscious waves of influence around them in so many ways, that reverberate through their environment and to those who come into contact with them.

By moving into harmony with nature, we enrich ourselves beyond measure. The happy person is not the one with the most possessions, or who can satisfy his every whim or who has a quick and easy "answer" to every problem. A selfless, harmonious person, whether he is a member of a primitive tribe or has all the riches of modern life, is the happier one.

Knowledge of your body and its fertility cycle is a step into a circle of harmony. It is another aspect of a wholesome and happy life. We hope you will take that step.

The Final Word

During the few months between completing this book and receiving the final proofs before printing, a number of factors have emerged from recent research findings. These may be summarized, as follows:

The Temperature Shift – A New Rule

A new rule is now proposed and taught by Dr Anna Flynn and the research team at Birmingham Maternity Hospital. This now reads:

The post-ovulatory phase begins on the third morning of a sustained temperature shift, all three of which are higher than ALL of the previous undisturbed temperatures, with the exception of the first four. The shift should be at least 0.2°C or 0.4°F between the last lower temperature and the highest of the next three.

The net result in the vast majority of cases is identical, but this method is more versatile in identifying the *biphasic* nature of a chart with a temperature shift, especially when there are small temperature fluctuations on a daily basis, even as the temperature is rising. As always, if in doubt, wait for the chart to clarify itself. This change does not affect *OVIA,* which uses a different mathematical set of rules to identify the shift. These rules are, after all, quite empirical – designed as close to 100% as possible of the ways in which a temperature shift can manifest. You may use either rule, but always be sure that you have found a true temperature shift, especially if you have a pattern of variable BBT recordings. You may find that one rule works better for your particular pattern than the other, in identifying the shift, when seen retrospectively.

An Extra Temperature Shift When Pregnant

When conception has taken place, there seems to be a second, upwards temperature shift, maybe only five or six days after the first shift. This is probably due to the increased level of progesterone after a successful fertilization and implantation. This additional shift is the earliest objective indicator of pregnancy.

Ovulation Pain or Mittelschmerz

It is becoming clear that in those women who consistently experience this pain (see page 28), it can be used almost as a major indicator. To incorporate it into the system of rules, you add four days, just as with Peak Mucus or the peak cervix indication, to calculate the start of the post-ovulatory infertile phase. Then you take the latest of all the indicators you are monitoring

Coming Off The Pill

The post-ovulatory or *luteal* phase of a cycle is normally between ten and sixteen days. When coming off the Pill, however, do not be surprised if this phase is reduced to less than ten days. If you are coming off the Pill and wanting to learn Natural Fertility Awareness, then it is really advisable to get individual tuition, just as it is even otherwise.

The broad guidelines are that you should always finish a complete pack of pills, taking the first day of the withdrawal bleed as the first day of the cycle, even though it is not a true period. You should chart the first cycle, but it cannot be regarded as safe at any time. There is also likely to be a divergence of indications, especially with copious mucus for much of the time to begin with, since you will have a excess of oestrogen in your system. As we said in the main text, take four days of temperature shift and generally overestimate on the safe side until cycles become normal. This will usually be within three to six cycles, depending also on the Pill that was in use. There are generally less of these problems when coming off the progesterone only, Mini-Pill.

Fertility Awareness and the IUCD

The presence of an IUCD normally increases the flow of mucus, due to the irritation caused within the uterus by the IUCD itself and to the cervix by the coil threads. Charting can begin before the removal of the IUCD and the normal biphasic temperature pattern should be observable. Cervix observations should be made, if possible, because the mucus pattern will be obscured and you can derive some natural benefit from the coil by using its string to guide you to the cervix.

So basically, learn to make your own observations before removal of the device, but have it removed as soon as possible after that. Then follow the same rules as for the Pill until normal cycles are resumed. If you can't stand the idea of it being in there any longer, then have it removed anyway.

Fertility Awareness after Childbirth

There are still no rules that can be applied to everyone after childbirth, because there are so many variable factors. However, the following guidelines represent our current knowledge.

1. **In a mother who is fully breastfeeding,** with the baby receiving no other food or drink, and being nursed at least every three hours:

   Infertility can be assured for the first five weeks.

   In fact, as long as the vaginal sensation remains dry you can be sure of continuing infertility. This infertile phase may last for as long as ten weeks. **Charting, however, should begin after five weeks**, and it is important to realise that ovulation can occur *before* the first the first menstruation. In addition, making matters a little confusing, there is often an extended period of moistness or wetness during the post-childbirth infertile phase, not necessarily associated with returning fertility. Finally, it is occasionally possible for women in their twelfth week of full lactation to be both ovulating and subsequently menstruating, so although ecological or full breastfeeding will inhibit the return of fertility, it does vary from person to person. The only rules that can be set, therefore, must take into account the earliest that ovulation has been known to occur, though in many cases the infertile phase wil continue for some longer period. It is worth mentioning that breastfeeding still remains the largest single factor in the world responsible for the spacing of children.

Part of the key to this pattern probably lies in the inhibitory effect on the fertility cycle of the lactation stimulating pituitary hormone, *prolactin*. Production of this hormone is stimulated by suckling and the general closeness between the mother and child.

2. **Partially breast feeding mothers** can expect ovulation as early as the twenty-seventh day (nearly four weeks). Taking the lifetime of sperm into account, this means that:

A period of infertility can be assured for only three weeks.

3. Similarly, a **mother who is artificially feeding her child,** can expect that:

Infertility can be assured for about three weeks.

In both cases, therefore, **charting should begin after three weeks**.

4. **During pregnancy,**the BBT remains high. After childbirth, it remains high to begin with, due probably to the effect of prolactin, but later it falls, indicating the gradual return of fertility. Ovulation is then followed by a normal temperature shift and menstruation.
5. There is a tendency for a woman's post-childbirth fertility pattern to repeat itself with successive babies, assuming that the children are raised identically.

International Correspondence Course

A thorough and comprehensive **Correspondence Course** has now been written and organised and is available from the **Natural Fertility Awareness Education Centre**, run by the Wholistic Research Company – please consult the last page for their address. This is designed to train both users and those who also wish to teach the methods to others – the network of teachers of these methods is now rapidly expanding.

Glossary

Please consult the index and the text for a full understanding of the subjects described below.

Abstinence	Voluntary avoidance of sexual intercourse.
Amenorrhea	Prolonged periods without menstruation.
Anovulatory Cycle	A menstrual cycle in which no ovulation occurs and which is therefore infertile.
Basal Body Temperature	The body temperature at rest, undisturbed by activity, food or drink. Normally, this means upon waking. It is affected by the hormone, progesterone, rising by about 0.2° C/0.4° F after ovulation has taken place. One of the three major indicators of natural fertility awareness.
Birth Control	A method of avoiding, achieving or spacing pregnancies in sexually active couples. Only natural methods can be used to achieve a pregnancy.
Breast Feeding	The natural method by which a baby receives love and nourishment directly from the mother's breasts, in the form of milk. This can be a complete source of food and drink or may be supplemented.
Breakthrough Bleeding	The small and occasional blood-stained discharge during the middle of a men-

strual cycle associated with the thickening and preparedness of the endometrium for a potential pregnancy. Also called *spotting* or *mid-cycle bleeding*.

Cervical Mucus — The fluid secreted by the cells lining the interior of the neck of the womb, the cervix. Its properties are affected by the hormones oestrogen and progesterone. It can be hostile or friendly to sperm survival and passage, depending upon the closeness to ovulation. One of the three major indicators of natural fertility awareness.

Cervical Os — The opening in the cervix that leads into the vagina.

Cervix — The lower end of the uterus that projects downwards into the vagina. Its properties change throughout the cycle, becoming one of the three major indicators of natural fertility awareness.

Climacteric — The time in a woman's life when her reproductive capability is declining.

Conception — The meeting and fusion of the ovum with a sperm and subsequent implantation in the uterine wall.

Contraception — See *Birth Control*.

Corpus Luteum — The body formed by the ovarian follicle after the release of the ovum. The hormone progesterone is secreted.

Cover Line — The line drawn on a chart to help identify the temperature shift between six lower and three higher temperatures.

Ectopic Pregnancy — An implantation of a fertilized ovum outside the uterus, normally in the Fallopian Tube.

Ejaculation	The emission of semen from the penis during a male orgasm.
Endocrine Gland	A gland that produces one or more hormones.
Endometrium	The wall of the uterus which is cyclically prepared to receive a fertilized ovum and subsequently shed at menstruation if pregnancy does not occur.
Fallopian Tube	The two tubes which extend from the upper uterus to the ovaries and through which the ovum travels on its way to meet the sperm. Fertilization normally takes place at the ovarian end of these tubes.
Family Planning	See *Birth Control*.
Fertile Phase	The time during the early part of a menstrual cycle before and around ovulation, when conception could take place.
Fertilization	The union of the ovum and the sperm.
Fertility Cycle	The waxing and waning of potential in a woman's reproductive system to become pregnant.
Hormones	Crucial chemical triggers controlling and administering physiological processes. The state of their balance has far reaching effects on anatomical, physiological, emotional and mental well-being and health.
Infertile Phase	The time during the very early and post-ovulatory phase of a menstrual cycle, when conception cannot occur.
Labia	The two sets of lips at the entrance to the vagina.
Menarche	The first menstruation in the life of a young woman.

Menopause	The last menstruation in the life of a woman.
Menstrual Cycle	The cyclic changes in a woman's reproductive system.
Menstruation	The cyclic shedding of the endometrium, consisting of blood, mucus and cellular material.
Metabolism	The physiological processes of building up and breaking down bodily tissues.
Mucus	See *Cervical Mucus*.
Natural Family Planning (NFP)	Natural methods of birth control. See *Birth Control*.
Natural Fertility Awareness	The natural awareness of the indicators which let a woman know of the fertile and infertile phases of her menstrual cycle.
Oestrogen	The female hormone produced by the ovaries during the fertile phase of a cycle.
Ovarian Follicle	The envelope of tissue containing the ovum that develops within the ovary. Also called the *Graafian Follicle*.
Ovaries	The two organs that produce the ova and female sex hormones.
Ovulation	The release of a mature ovum from an *Ovarian Follicle*.
Ovum	The female egg, ready for fertilization. Plural: ova.
Pregnancy (human)	The implantation of a fertilized ovum and its growth into a baby, born usually about nine months later.
Progesterone	The hormone secreted by the Corpus Luteum controlling the post-ovulatory phase of the menstrual cycle and early pregnancy.

Puberty	The onset of mature sexual function. Associated with changes in both primary and secondary sexual characteristics.
Scrotum	The sack of skin holding and protecting the testes.
Seminal Vesicle	The two sperm-storage sacs. They also supply nutrition and fluid to the sperm.
Sperm	The male reproductive or germ cell.
Spotting	See *Breakthrough Bleeding.*
Testes	The male organs producing sperm and male hormones responsible for developing and maintaining the secondary male sexual characteristics.
Testosterone	A male hormone produced by the testes, maintaining the secondary male sexual characteristics.
Uterus	The womb or cavity-shaped muscular organ in which the fertilized ovum is implanted and develops.
Vagina	The muscular, cavity-shaped organ that extends from the opening to the outside world (the vulva) to the cervix.
Vaginal Discharge	Fluid or other material coming from the vaginal walls, which may or may not be normal. Cervical mucus and menstrual discharge pass *through* the vagina, but are not vaginal discharge.
Vas Deferens	The narrow tubes through which the sperm is transferred to the seminal vesicles.
Vulva	The opening of the vagina to the outside world, being made up of two sets of lips (*labia majors* and *minora*) and the *clitoris.*

Bibliography and Further Reading

Natural Fertility Awareness

The Art of Natural Family Planning, John and Sheila Kippley; The Couple to Couple League, 1984.

The Billings Method, Dr. Evelyn Billings and Ann Westmore; O'Donovan, 1980, Australia.

Electro-metric Timing of Human Ovulation, L. Langman and H. S. Burr; American Journal of Obstetrics and Gynaecology. 44, 1942.

Lunaception, Louise Lacey; Warner, New York, 1976.

A Manual of Natural Family Planning, Dr. Anna Flynn and Melissa Brooks; Allen and Unwin, 1984.

*Natural Family Planning,*Professor John Marshall; Catholic Marriage Advisory Council, 1978.

On the Possibility of a Perfect Rhythm Method of Birth Control by Periodic Light Stimulation, E. M. Dewan; American Journal of Obstetrics & Gynaecology, 99(7), 1967.

Unnatural Birth Control

Amenorrhoea Following Oral Contraception, J. R. Evrard & al.; American Journal of Obstetrics and Gynaecology, 124, 1976.

The Birth Control Book, Howard I. Shapiro; Penguin, 1980.

Detailed Leaflet on Labelling and Information To Be Supplied with Contraceptives, Food and Drug Administration, United States; April 1978.

Oral and Intrauterine Contraception: a 1978 Risk Assessment, A. Rosenfield; American Journal of Obstetrics and Gynecology, 132, 1978.

The Which? Guide to Birth Control, Penny Kane; Consumers' Association, 1983.

Women and the Crisis in Sex Hormones, B. and G. Seaman; Rawson Associates, New York, 1977.

Infertility

Childlessness: Its Causes and What To Do About Them, Elliot Philip; Arrow, 1975.

Coping with Childlessness, Diane and Peter Houghton; Allen and Unwin, 1984.

The Experience of Infertility, Naomi Pfeffer and Anne Woollet; Virago, 1983.

Factsheets, National Association For The Childless.

The Fertility Question, Margaret Nofziger; The Book Publishing Company, 1982.

Infertile Marriage, Robert Newill; Harmondsworth: Penguin, 1974.

Infertility, Consumers' Association, 1972.

Why Us?, Dr. Andrew Stanway; Thorsons, 1984.

Women's Cycles

Female Cycles, Paula Weideger; The Woman's Press, 1975.

The Wise Wound: Menstruation and Every Woman, Penelope Shuttle and Peter Redgrove; Gollancz, 1978.

Menopause

Menopause: A Positive Approach, Rosetta Reitz; Allen and Unwin, 1977.

General

Blueprint for Immortality, Harold S. Burr; Spearman, 1972.

The Cycles of Heaven, Guy Lyon Playfair and Scott Hill; Souvenir, 1978.

Green Pharmacy, Barbara Griggs. Norman and Hobhouse, 1982.

Secrets of A Coral Island, Bob Johannes; BBC 2 film, November 29th, 1976.

Further Information

Further reading and information on the subjects discussed in this book, as well as fertility charts, thermometers, OVUSTICK and *OVIA*, plus an:

INTERNATIONAL CORRESPONDENCE COURSE

on the personal use and teaching of

NATURAL FERTILITY AWARENESS

are all available from:

Natural Fertility Awareness Education Centre,
Wholistic Research Company
Bright Haven, Robin's Lane, Lolworth,
Cambridge CB3 8HH, England.
Telephone: Crafts Hill (0954) 81074

Please send them two first class stamps if you are living within the United Kingdom. Agent and distributor enquiries are welcome.

Index